The

4 Steps

of
Long Term Care Planning

Susan B. Day
Thomas Day

Published by the

National Care Planning Council
P.O. Box 1118
Centerville, UT 84014
800-989-8137

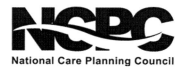

National Care Planning Council

www.longtermcarelink.net
CONTACT: inquiry@longtermcarelink.net

ISBN: 978-0-9816827-2-3

Quantities of this book are available at special discounts for bulk purchases, for sales promotions, premiums, fundraising or educational use by members of the National Care Planning Council. Special discounts are also available for book resellers and libraries. Call the number above. You can also order this book online at www.4stepsbook.com.

Cover designed by Misty Day

Printed by DMT publishing, North Salt Lake, Utah
www.dmtpublishing.com
October 2007
Revised April 8, 2008

TABLE OF CONTENTS

STEP 2 - Funding the Cost of Long Term Care 39

II

STEP 3 - Using Long Term Care Professionals 79

STEP 4 - Creating a Personal Care Plan and Choosing a Care Coordinator

INTRODUCTION

Planning for the Elder Years

If we were to ask an older person what his or her most important concerns for aging are, we would probably get a variety of different answers. According to surveys frequently conducted among the elderly, the most likely answers we would receive would include the following three principal concerns or life wishes:

1. Remaining independent in the home without intervention from others
2. Maintaining good health and receiving adequate health care
3. Having enough money for everyday needs and not outliving assets and income.

To address these concerns or wishes and maintain the quality of life wanted in the elder years, it simply takes a little preplanning.

It is human nature not to worry about an event until it happens.

We may prepare financially for unexpected financial disasters by covering our homes, automobiles and health with insurance policies. But no other life event can be as devastating to an elderly person's lifestyle, finances and security as needing long term care. It drastically alters or completely eliminates the three principal lifestyle wishes listed above.

It is our experience that the majority of the American public does not plan for this crisis of needing eldercare. The lack of planning also has an adverse effect on the older person's family, with sacrifices made in time, money, and family lifestyles.

Because of changing demographics and potential changes in government funding, the current generation needs to plan for long term care before the elder years are upon them.

Let us look at some facts.

- The population of the "very old," -- older than age 85 -- is the fastest growing group in America. This population is at highest risk for needing care. (*Statistical abstract of the United States, 2005 , population*)
- Medical science is preventing early sudden deaths, which means living longer with impaired health and greater risk of needing long term care.
- The Alzheimer's Association estimates the risk of Alzheimer's or dementia beyond age 85 to be about 46% of that population.
- It is estimated that 6 out of 10 people will need long term care sometime during their lifetime.
- Children are moving far away from parents or parents move away during retirement making long distance care giving difficult or impossible.
- Government programs -- already stretched thin for long term care services -- will experience even greater stress on available funds in the future.

Below are some excuses we have heard from people who refuse to plan for long term care. Some of these objections may seem perfectly reasonable, but are still excuses and not actually what happens. In fact, the opposite outcome of these excuses is often the case.

"I'm in good health and will live a long time, and I won't need it."
"No one in my family has ever needed it."
"My family has a history of early deaths and poor health. I'll die first."
"Aunt Nellie is 100 years old and doing great." (Forgot to mention she is in a nursing home)
"I'm a veteran and the VA will take care of me."
"I will have the government pay for it."
"My kids say they will take care of me."
"My daughter is a nurse. She will take care of me."
"I'm too busy right now. I'll do something in the future."
"I'm not worried. When the time comes, I'll deal with it."

Education on long term care and resources available is critical to preparing and planning for eldercare. For example, a person with the actual knowledge of the VA program will know that there has to be a medical need and that the veteran must have a substantial service-connected disability or have a very low income before VA will furnish long term care services.

Or for example, saying government Medicaid will cover you is saying that you will be impoverished. In order to qualify for Medicaid you must have less than $2,000 in assets and income insufficient to pay the cost of care.

One of the important things to plan for is how to maintain your lifestyle as you age. You may be healthy enough to stay in your own home, with help provided for the following activities of daily living: maintaining a home, providing meals, supervision, companionship, transportation and shopping services.

But, this type of home care is non-medical and must be provided free of charge by family, friends, or volunteers or the care must be paid for out-of-pocket by the family. Government programs, in most cases, will not pay for this kind of care. It is estimated that 80% of all long term care is non-medical, with 90% of that care provided in the home. It is most likely that your long term care will begin with home care.

The process of long-term care planning involves the following four principles:

1. Knowledge and preparation are the keys to success.
2. Having funds to pay for care expands the choices for care settings and providers.
3. Using professional help relieves stress, reduces conflict, and saves time and money.
4. Success is assured through a written plan accepted by all parties involved.

Our purpose in this book is to dispel the myths, correct the misconception of what government programs offer, and educate the public on every aspect of planning for long term care.

Using our experience, research, and education in all areas of long term, we have filled the pages of this book with needed information, resources, and guidance to help you create a long term care plan that fits your lifestyle and financial situation. Or if you are planning for a loved one, the resources and instructions in our book will help alleviate the stress and the burden on you of trying to provide that care

STEP 1

Understanding the Nature of Care, Care Settings, and Government Programs

Knowledge and preparation are the keys to success.

What is Long Term Care and Eldercare?

Long term care and eldercare are synonymous as far as services provided. The difference is a person of any age can receive long term care; whereas, only the elderly receive eldercare.

Long term care refers to a broad range of supportive medical, personal, and social services needed by people who are unable to meet their basic living needs for an extended period of time. This need for care may be caused by an accident, illness, or frailty. Such conditions may require help with the ability to move about, dress, bathe, eat, use a toilet, medicate, and avoid incontinence.

Also care may be needed to help the disabled person with household cleaning, preparing meals, shopping, paying bills, visiting the doctor, answering the phone, and taking medications.

Oftentimes, long term care in the form of constant supervision, is needed due to cognitive impairment from stroke, depression, dementia, Alzheimer's, Parkinson's, and so on.

Long term care requires a healthy person to provide support for the disabled person. This support can be offered at home or in a facility. As a rule those who are disabled prefer to stay at home and, most of the time so-called informal caregivers (family and friends) prefer the home as well; however, the deciding factor of where to receive help ultimately centers on the nature of the disability. For example, a wife caring for her overweight husband may be unable to help him bathe, dress, use the toilet, or even transfer from the bed to a chair. She will either have to hire aides to come to the home or put him in a facility.

Another example might be an Alzheimer's patient who has become unmanageable and must receive constant supervision. This may be impossible at home and an Alzheimer's facility may be the only solution.

Understanding the Need and Setting for Long Term Care
The need for long term care may only last for a few weeks or months or it may go on for years. It all depends on the underlying reasons for needing care.

Temporary Long Term Care (need for care only weeks or months)
- Rehabilitation from a hospital stay
- Recovery from illness
- Recovery from injury
- Recovery from surgery
- Terminal medical condition

Ongoing Long Term Care (need for care many months or years)

- Chronic medical conditions
- Chronic severe pain
- Permanent disabilities
- Dementia
- Ongoing need for help with activities of daily living
- Need for supervision

Long term care services may be provided in any of the following settings:

- In the home of the recipient
- In the home of a family member or friend of the recipient

- At an adult day services location
- In an assisted living facility or board-and-care home
- In a hospice facility
- In a nursing home

Custodial Care versus Skilled Care

Custodial care and skilled care are terms used by the medical community and health care plans such as health insurance companies, Medicare, Medicaid and the Veterans Administration. They are used primarily to differentiate long term care provided by medical specialists as opposed to care provided by aides, volunteers, family, or friends.

The use of these terms and their application is important in determining whether a health care plan will pay for long term care services or not. Generally, skilled services are paid for by a health care plan and custodial services, not in conjunction with skilled care, are not covered. However, custodial services are almost always a part of a skilled service plan of care and, by being included; custodial services are paid by the health care plan as well. Many people have the misconception that only skilled services are covered. This is simply not true.

According to the American College of Medical Quality:

> **"Skilled care** is the provision of services and supplies that can be given only by or under the supervision of skilled or licensed medical personnel.
> **Custodial care** is the provision of services and supplies that can be given safely and reasonably by individuals who are neither skilled nor licensed medical personnel."

The terms skilled and custodial refer to the people who deliver the care, not the actual care given.

A skilled care provider can also provide services normally thought to be provided by custodial caregivers. Such things as help with activities of daily living and so-called instrumental activities of daily living are often furnished by skilled providers in the course of their treatment. Or a skilled care plan may call for services that can be delivered by a custodial caregiver, but it would still be under the skilled plan of care for that individual. On the other hand, people who deliver custodial services may from time to time perform those activities supposedly reserved for skilled providers. Such things as taking blood pressure, supervising medicines, preparing shots, or changing wounds might be provided under certain circumstances by a custodial provider.

Formal Care versus Informal Care

Formal Caregivers
Formal caregivers are volunteers or paid care providers associated with a service system. Service systems might include for-profit or nonprofit nursing homes, intermediate care facilities, assisted living, home care agencies, community services, hospice, church or charity service groups, adult day care, senior centers, association services, state aging services, and so on.

Informal Caregivers
Informal caregivers are family, friends, neighbors, or church members who provide unpaid care out of love, respect, obligation, or friendship to a disabled person. These people far outnumber formal caregivers, and without them this country would have a difficult time providing funding for the caregiving needs of a growing number of long term care recipients.

Depending on the definition of caregiving, estimates of the number of informal caregivers range from 20 million to 50 million people. This could represent about 20% of the total population providing part-time or full-time care for loved ones.

About two-thirds of those caregivers for people over age 50 are employed full-time or part-time and two-thirds of those–about 45% of all working caregivers–report having to rearrange their work schedule, decrease their hours or take an unpaid leave in order to meet their caregiving responsibilities.

The average amount of time informal caregivers provide assistance is 4.5 years, but 20% will provide care for 5 years or longer. (National long term care survey 1999)

Understanding the Progression of Care Commitment
The chart below illustrates the relationship of informal care to formal care. As care needs increase, both in the number of hours required and in the number or intensity of activities requiring help, there is a greater need for the services of formal caregivers. Unfortunately, many informal caregivers become so focused on their task, they don't realize they are getting in over their heads and that they have reached the point where partial or total formal caregiving is necessary. Or the informal caregiver may recognize the need for paid, professional help but does not have the money to pay for it.

Depending on what causes the need for long term care, a care-recipient could start out at any point on the curve below. For instance, a stroke, injury, or sudden illness may result in the immediate need for part time or full time care. On the other hand, the slowly progressing infirmity of old age, the slow onset of dementia, or a progressively deteriorating medical condition may only require occasional help; beginning with intermittent care from an informal caregiver but gradually progressing to the need for full time, formal care.

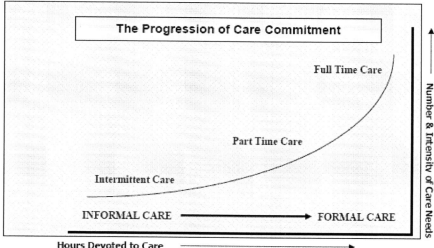

Making a Plan for Your Long Term Care

Very few people plan for the eldercare or long term care part of their lifes, but planning for care is as important, if not more important than their retirement plan. If we do not plan, we are leaving our last years in someone else's hands. In the following example we see that as much as our children love us and mean to do right by us, they cannot possibly know what we want if they are not told.

Ruby, age 80, lost her husband. She had cared for him at home after his stroke. Understandably, she felt lost and depressed after his death. An inner ear infection caused Ruby to lose her balance, and she fell, breaking her hip. While she was in the hospital, recuperating from surgery, Ruby's children were deciding her future.

Concerned for her health and safety, they moved some of her belongings to an assisted care facility. Upon Ruby's release from the hospital, she was taken to her new home at the facility. Between pain medication and the unfamiliar surroundings, Ruby never was herself again. She spent her last days asking what had happened to her home and items in it that meant so much to her. Though her children had her best interest at heart, they did not know how Ruby wanted to spend her elder days.

An article on the AARP website titled, "Talking about Independent Living" states,

"Research has shown that, as people age, they prefer to continue living independently, preferably in their own homes. While adult children often worry about their parents' situation, it can be difficult to know if parents really need, or want, help from their children."

The article continues to suggest ways for children to talk to their parents about health, and finances, driving, taking medication, and living alone.

We agree whole-heartedly that children and parents should talk about all these things, except the parents should be the instigators and set the plan for the children to follow.

What do you want your children or friends to do in your behalf? When it comes time for them to help, you may not be physically or mentally able to execute your wishes. This is where your long term care plan comes into effect.

There is a lot to learn about long term care. A large amount of material is put out to help you with the decisions that need to be made. Learning what long term care is and how to qualify for Federal government aid or state services is very important. You may need a lot of care or a little. It may be home care, assisted living care, or nursing home care.

Reasons to make your plan now

- Avoid the mistakes of parents
- Reduce the future burden on family members
- Provide funding in advance
- Complete estate planning
- Make wishes known in advance
- Provide advance medical directives
- Provide financial information
- Provide an inheritance in advance for family members
- Provide training on whom to contact for help

Finding Help for Current Caregiving Needs for Loved Ones
Long term care planning can also be useful for older people who failed to plan when they were younger. These people will likely be forced to rely on Medicaid for their care. Making a plan offers strategies to lessen the financial and emotional impact on potential Medicaid recipients and their families. Going through the four steps of planning can help you make the best decisions for their care.

Immediate Planning Needs
- Handling the care crisis for family caregivers
- Education on caregiving options
- Determining how best to handle financial costs
- Determining desires or wishes of your elder parent
- Knowing where to turn for help

Understanding Care Settings

Considering where you want to live at the time of retirement is a big factor in your long term care plan. At retirement, your health may be good and consideration of long term care needs in the future is easily disregarded at this time; when, in fact, this is the best time to develop a plan. Plans should be centered on remaining at home as long as possible.

The chart below puts into perspective the number and types of senior living arrangements at the end of the year 2000. By far, the majority of older adults are remaining in their homes or in the homes of their families.

Estimates of senior living arrangements in the United States at the end of the year 2000.	total numbers	percent of total age 65+ population
U.S. population age 65 and older	34,992,000	100.0%
Age 65 and older owning and living in their own homes	27,434,000	78.4%
Age 65 and older renting, living with family or other	2,976,000	8.5%
Available assisted living beds	1,706,000	4.9%
Age 65 and older residents living in nursing homes	1,475,000	4.2%
Available seniors apartments	821,000	2.3%
Available independent living community beds	239,000	0.7%
Available continuing care retirement community beds	171,000	0.5%
Available units, combined care communities	171,000	0.5%

Census information was derived from the national census online. Seniors owning their own homes and age 65 and over nursing home residents were taken from the 2003, Statistical Abstract Of The United States. All other data were derived from the following source:
"The NIC National Supply Estimate of Seniors Housing & Care Properties

Whether you are considering selling your home and purchasing a retirement home, renting an apartment, moving to an assisted living community, or staying in your current home, these choices determine the type of care options you put into your plan.

Below are listed some of the living arrangements available for seniors. We also note whether they have long term care available as well as financial help.

Retirement Communities

Retirement communities are very popular with people 55 and older. Many of these communities are built in resort areas where climates are warmer. Community living arrangements typically include recreational amenities for the elderly. In contemplating a move, it may be wise to consider retirement communities that have the availability of care services, should the need arise in the future.

Some retirement communities provide what might be called supportive care. This might be help in the form of prepared meals, housekeeping services, transportation, planned events, and reminder services.

Master Planned Active Adult Communities

Adult communities are often called by descriptive names such as "resort community", "golf community", or "adult retirement community". These master planned communities are developed specifically for people over certain prescribed ages such as age 55, age 62, or age 65. At least one member of the household must meet the age restriction. These arrangements almost always offer individual, owner-occupied units. The appeal of these communities is to offer active seniors, selling their existing house, to trade equity from the old home into a newer, attractive unit about the same size or larger.

This housing varies from simple apartments to high rise condominiums to single family detached housing. Costs range from a low of $25,000 (800 sq. ft. manufactured home) to well over $500,000. Some communities are upscale exclusively and may cater only to high income seniors.

Planned Communities with No Age Restrictions

Seniors who do not want to live in a structured adult retirement community may choose a Planned Unit Development that contains several sizes and options of dwellings and has no age restrictions. A PUD gives them the opportunity to live in a mixed-age neighborhood, perhaps in a more secure area, where some of the headaches of home ownership -- such as yard care -- have been removed.

Purchasing costs of a dwelling in a Planned Unit Development vary from type and size of the structure, as well as location. Generally cost is equivalent to current real estate prices in the area.

Condominiums

A condominium, or condo as it is commonly called, is a form of ownership and not a development plan. However, a condo project may be part of a planned community as well. The owner of a condo unit has title to all of the interior airspace and the interior walls, ceilings and floors of the dwelling unit. The rest of the superstructure including the exterior, the land, and all of the amenities belong to all the other condominium owners as common property.

The advantage of owning a condo is that the dwelling space is solely owned and not a rental, thereby allowing the owner to carry a mortgage that would someday be paid off. Or the owner may elect to pay cash and never have to make payments again. Senior-only condominium projects are available.

 Purchasing costs would be consistent with real estate in your area.

Manufactured Housing Communities (Mobile Home Parks)

A growing number of manufactured housing communities own the land comprising the community on a cooperative basis. Cooperative ownership gives manufactured home residents control over management and operating costs of the park, while owning a manufactured home of their own. In these communities, you will be renting the lot for the manufactured home you own.

> Ownership in retirement communities, master-plan adult communities, condominiums and manufactured housing, as well as staying in your currently owned home, provides the following advantages for future long term care needs.
> - Financial benefits: home equity loan, reverse mortgage, cash from sale of property
> - Long term care benefits and services: Option to remain living in your own home and paying for home care services as needed.

Seniors Apartments

Seniors only apartments allow seniors to rent in a community with people their own age. Senior renters may be individuals who have owned a home or have been renting all of their life but desire to move to a community that supports a senior lifestyle.

Senior apartments can vary in terms of services but typically offer apartment living and services designed specifically for independent active seniors 55 and older. Senior apartment complexes are usually located near senior centers, parks, shopping malls, golf courses, and public transportation. Many offer van services along with monthly road trips to shows and casinos.

Independent Living Facilities and Congregate Housing

Independent living or congregate housing communities are residential communities for older adults who want an enjoyable lifestyle free of the worries and trouble of home maintenance. They are similar to apartment, condominium, or single-family developments except that they provide special services, including security—an important consideration for many residents.

Most independent living communities are fully secured; staff members greet and screen all visitors around the clock. Residents can leave home for extended periods of time knowing that their living quarters will be safe.

Many of these communities provide housing to people with lower income and as a result, often lack the amenities of communities discussed previously. Some of these communities also provide government rent subsidies for very low income residents.

Another difference between this living arrangement and those discussed previously is there is often more accommodation made for care. These communities may offer linen services, maid service, handyman help, meal programs, transportation and even help in getting around the facility as long as it doesn't require a major commitment from the staff.

In many respects these communities are similar to assisted living except assisted living also is licensed to provide additional care services such as help with bathing, dressing, toileting, diapering, medicating, help with daily living decisions, and help with moving from one place to another. Some independent living communities accommodate care needs by providing access to home health services from an independent agency.

Senior apartment and independent or congregate living facilities provide the following options for long term care:
- Financial benefits: No significant financial benefits for long term care. You are paying rent or monthly fees and do not own property.
- Long term care benefits: Some assistance and aid as well as security. Home care if needed will be paid by you.

Assisted Living Facilities

Assisted living is exactly as it says. Living in an apartment or facility where you receive assistance with daily personal needs. Residents remain independent while receiving assistance as needed with personal care, medications, transportation, housekeeping, meals, and other daily living needs.

Assisted living facilities offer a less expensive and often more desirable arrangement to a nursing home. They are designed for those people who have some care needs, but don't have the physical, medical, or mental impairments that require a nursing home.

Assisted living definitions vary from state to state. Each state has its own licensing requirements and regulations for these types of facilities. Thus they may be titled differently and offer varying degrees and types of services depending on state law.

The structure of assisted living facilities can range from a dwelling that looks like a home in a residential area where the caregiver is the owner and single proprietor, to a large, apartment-style building staffed with many employees. The care style is different in these two examples.

A board-and-care in a residential area, with three to eight beds provides a homelike environment and closer association with the other residents. Each resident has his or her own room and bathroom. Living room and dining areas are commonly shared with other residents. With little support staff, you need to be mobile enough to get yourself around, and other services may be limited.

In contrast, large assisted living facilities may be staffed with 24 hour nursing care, a help desk, entertainment, and educational programs and provide large private apartments. Arrangements are sometimes made for home health agencies, therapists, or visiting doctors for residents' needs. Transportation, excursions and field trips are also available.

No matter the size, assisted living facilities offer individual choices, independence, and security of not being alone.

When choosing to move to an assisted living facility, you should look to the future at what your needs might be. If you move to a smaller, board-and-care facility and you develop a medical condition that requires more care than it can give, you will be looking at another move to get that care. If you do prefer the individual home concept, check to see if home care medical assistance can come in to aid you when needed.

The cost of assisted living facilities varies with the type of facility and the services given. In most cases you will pay a regular monthly rent which will include meals and housekeeping. Services beyond that may be charged separately. Costs and services also vary from state to state because there are states that allow only limited services and some that even allow full nursing home care in assisted living facilities.

Some facilities provide levels of care based on need, and charges are uniform for each level. For instance level 1 may cost an additional $400 a month and level 2 might cost $800 for more a month.

Long term care insurance will cover all or part of assisted living costs. This includes care costs and room and board. All modern comprehensive long term care insurance policies cover assisted living upon meeting the qualifying requirements.

Medicaid -- if it pays at all -- typically will only pay for "care costs" and not for room and board. Care costs include things like help with bathing, dressing, incontinence, medications, and nursing needs. Medicaid qualifications must be met. Medicare does not pay for assisted living.

For the most part, assisted living is paid for by personal funds.

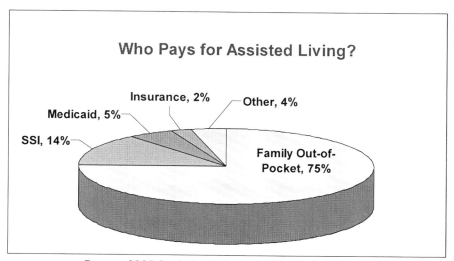

Who Pays for Assisted Living?

- Insurance, 2%
- Other, 4%
- Medicaid, 5%
- SSI, 14%
- Family Out-of-Pocket, 75%

Source: 2005 Statistical Abstract of the United States

Continuing Care Retirement Communities
Continuing care retirement communities -- sometimes called life care communities -- have been around for over 30 years. These are

typically exclusive upscale retirement complexes for people with a sizable down payment such as $200,000 and the ability to pay monthly fees of anywhere from $1,500-$3,000. They are almost exclusively built and maintained by nonprofit corporations or religious organizations.

The original concept for CCRCs was to guarantee the residents a permanent retirement living arrangement where they would never have to move. If the need for care in one of these communities were to arise, the community would furnish, at no additional cost, home care, assisted living or nursing home care.

Unfortunately, the escalating cost of long term care services has made it impossible for many of these communities to guarantee long term care at no additional cost. Services are still available, but in many of these communities the residents must pay additional out-of-pocket for long term care.

Combined Care Communities
These communities combine independent living, assisted living, and a nursing home within the same building or separate buildings in close proximity on the same campus. These communities do not require a sizable down payment, but they are generally not as fancy or exclusive as continuing care communities either. The combined care community may also own a home health agency as well, thus providing a full spectrum of care. There are several benefits to this arrangement.

1. As need for care progresses you can remain in the same facility to receive it.
2. If you have a spouse living with you, who needs more extended care, you both can remain together in the same place.
3. The facility will become your home with friendships and perhaps in an area close to family. Being able to remain in the same place as the need for care escalates, can be mentally and emotionally satisfying.

One example of choosing this type of retirement living arrangement is Gerald and his wife Kathy. In their late 60's, they wanted to sell their home and move to a retirement community. Their desire was to move where they would not have so much maintenance on a home and could enjoy social activities with other seniors. Another consideration in their move was Gerald's diabetes and Kathy's arthritis. Both were starting to have some physical problems from years of suffering with these illnesses. Living in a combined care community would give them the freedom they needed now with the security of assisted living available in the future.

Five years after making their move, Kathy suffered a severe stroke, making her need for care critical. It was determined that she needed the care in the nursing home section of the combined care campus. Gerald felt at this time, he would do better living in the assisted living building connected to the nursing home. There he would receive assistance with meals, medication, and other personal needs. He would be close to Kathy and could walk to her room often for visits.

The transition to different living arrangements to match the care they needed was quick and simple. There was very little change to adjust too and their friends in the retirement community were still close by.

Costs of living and care in these types of communities are comparable to assisted living and nursing homes. Long term care insurance may pay for all or part, depending on qualifications. Medicaid will pay for nursing home costs after asset spend down and income qualifications are met. Medicare does not pay for assisted living, but will pay some domiciled nursing home costs under certain circumstances.

Assisted living, continuing care retirement communities and combined care communities provide the following resources for long term care:
- Financial Benefits: Mostly out of pocket payment for rooms and services until a medical need may result in Medicaid funds. Long term care insurance may pay all or part depending on your policy requirements.
- Long Term Care Benefits: Assistive care, security, medical care and nursing care depending on facility.

Nursing Homes

Nursing homes provide a cost-effective way to enable patients with injuries; acute illnesses or postoperative care needs to recover in an environment outside a hospital. About 91% of the 1,650,000 US nursing home residents are over the age of 65.

Nursing homes serve two kinds of residents. The first are those who have been discharged from the hospital for rehabilitative care. Medicare pays for a limited time for this kind of nursing home care.

Second are residents who may suffer from a wide array of physical or mental disorders or they may simply be feeble and unable to move about, bath themselves, or provide their own meals. These are long term care residents. Medicare does not pay for their type of care, but if qualifications are met, Medicaid will pay these nursing home costs. These people are often referred to as "long term care" residents.

It is hard to determine the length of time a stay in a nursing home will be. It depends on if it is for temporary rehabilitation or long term care for something like dementia. According to the *1999 National Nursing Home Survey* the average length of stay for all residents is 2.44 years.

How Do You Select a Nursing Home for Long Term Care?

- Choice Made by Hospital Discharge Planner

You may not need nursing home care until after an illness or injury has sent you to the hospital for treatment. All hospitals have a discharge planning service. One responsibility of this planning service is to assess and arrange for post-hospital care if necessary. If the discharge planner determines a need for nursing home care, then he or she usually chooses the appropriate facility with consent of the patient and family. Your doctor also has to have visiting arrangements with the nursing home where you will be. The planner also arranges for Medicare.

As a prospective purchaser, you do not have to agree with or accept the planner's decision, and you can offer an alternative location if you feel more comfortable. The facility, however, has to be a skilled nursing provider and a staff doctor must be available on a 24-hour emergency basis. The facility must also have access to a hospital with emergency room treatment.

- Referral

Many nursing home admissions are not made directly from a hospital, so the potential resident, or more likely the family, must choose a facility among perhaps dozens in his area. Selection of the appropriate home is important, especially in light of the proliferation of abuse and neglect problems. A valuable resource is a good referral from friends or relatives who have had someone close to them in a nursing home. Make sure they are familiar with the quality of care in the facility they are recommending.

- Phone Survey

It's a good idea to call all the facilities in your area and ask for bed rates. Also ask about staff turnover; age of the facility; whether the rate includes extras such as diapers and personal items; whether it is a chain, locally owned or nonprofit, and whether they offer the level of care you need. You can eliminate a number of facilities before you take the next step of an inspection tour.

- Amenities Are Nice, But...

The newness of a facility and the amenities say nothing about the quality of care. Nor is a high daily bed rate always an indicator of better care. Many older facilities have lower fixed costs, and they may be able to give quality care at lower rates even if the surroundings are not so spiffy. The staff and administration are the key to a quality nursing home stay, not the physical surroundings. A good indicator of quality is how long staff members have been with the facility. Long tenures usually mean job satisfaction. These people probably enjoy working with residents and are likely to have a good rapport with their charges and dispense high quality care. Always ask about tenure and turnover rates.

- Inspection Tour

When possible, make visits at various times during the day to the nursing home you are interested in to make personal observations of the staff and residents.

- Checklists

There are numerous checklists and evaluation helps on the internet to assist you in the selection of a nursing home in your area.

Costs for Nursing Home Care

The cost of a nursing home depends a great deal on where it is located in the country and whether it charges more for private paying patients versus Medicaid and Medicare patients. The Internet is replete with nursing home search services and prices in any given area, with specific nursing homes, can easily be determined.

Nursing homes look very much like hospitals. Staff is housed in accessible nursing stations. Residents live in utilitarian, hospital-like rooms with little or no privacy, and they sleep on hospital beds and are usually referred to as "patients" by the staff. Hospital pricing models are also used. Residents are charged daily flat rates for semiprivate or private rooms just like a hospital. Extra services and supplies are added to the bill. This pricing model assumes that all residents require the same supervision and care. Of course this is not true.

Medicare Nursing Home Coverage

Traditional Medicare will pay for 20 days of a skilled nursing care facility at full cost and the difference between $128 per day (2008 rate) and the actual cost for another 80 days. Private Medicare supplement insurance usually pays the 80 day deductible of $128 per day. However, Medicare often stops paying before reaching the full 100 days. When Medicare stops, so does the supplement coverage.

To qualify for Medicare nursing home coverage, the individual must spend at least 3 full days in a hospital and must have a skilled nursing need and have a doctor order it. The transfer from a hospital must occur within a certain time period. The new Medicare Advantage Plans generally cover nursing homes differently from traditional Medicare. Most plans require payment upfront as opposed to traditional Medicare that pays 100% first.

There is a misconception that Medicare automatically covers up to 100 days of all nursing home stays. In reality, 100 full days of Medicare coverage is not that likely. When the skilled nursing need is not required, then Medicare stops paying.

Not all nursing home admissions come from a hospital--a prerequisite for Medicare coverage. Note from the chart below that less than half of all nursing home admissions are from the hospital. Also, a hospital stay resulting in nursing home care does not automatically qualify for Medicare coverage. The stay may have been less than 3 full days or there may not be a skilled need.

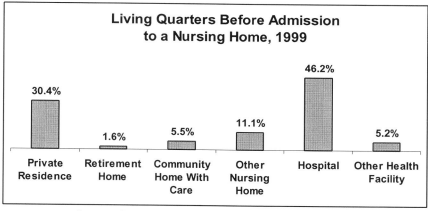

Source: 2005 statistical abstract of the United States

Medicaid
Medicaid is a welfare program, jointly funded by the federal government and the states and largely administered by the states. In 1998, Medicaid paid for 46.3% of the $88 billion received by all US nursing homes. To qualify for Medicaid a person must spend down his or her liquid assets to less than $2,000 and his or her monthly income must be insufficient to cover the cost of care. (*More details about Medicaid qualifications under STEP 2*)

Insurance
Insurance is an alternative source of funding for long term nursing home care. From virtually nothing in previous years, insurance paid 7.5% of nursing home receipts in 2002. This percentage is increasing every year.

The government is also sending a clear message it wants private insurance to play a larger role. This began with the recommendation of the Pepper Commission in 1992 and continued with the HIPAA legislation in 1996 and on to the offering in 2003 of long term care insurance for federal workers, military, retirees and their families.

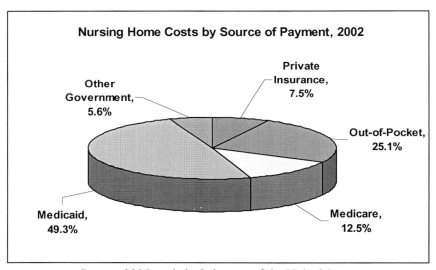

Source: 2005 statistical abstract of the United States

Home Care

Living In Your Home with Care Provided by Others
Long term care provided in the individual's home is the most preferable to the aging elderly. It is the type of caregiving that comes about naturally as the need for help with daily activities becomes necessary for one living in his or her own home. There are two types of home care providers: informal and formal.

Informal Caregivers

Informal caregivers are usually non-paid individuals who primarily provide home care and fulfill the needs of a disabled person. Family members are considered informal caregivers.

Home care is almost always provided in the home of the recipient or the home of a family member or friend. Home care may, under certain circumstances, be offered in other settings such as group homes or independent retirement communities. Below are some of the activities provided by or supervised by informal caregivers.

- Help with walking, lifting, and bathing
- Help with using the bathroom and with incontinence
- Providing pain management
- Preventing unsafe behavior and preventing wandering
- Providing comfort and assurance or arranging for professional counseling
- Feeding
- Answering the phone
- Making arrangements for therapy, meeting medical needs, and doctors' appointments
- Providing meals
- Maintaining the household
- Shopping and running errands
- Providing transportation
- Administering medications
- Managing money and paying bills
- Doing the laundry
- Attending to personal hygiene and personal grooming
- Writing letters or notes
- Making repairs to the home, maintaining a yard, and removing snow

Formal Caregivers

Formal caregivers are mostly paid care providers associated with a service system. Care is provided by home care companies, aging services, assisted living, hospice care and nursing homes.

More people are using informal and formal home care over community care or nursing home care. The chart below shows the average care setting and length of time for elderly over age 65.

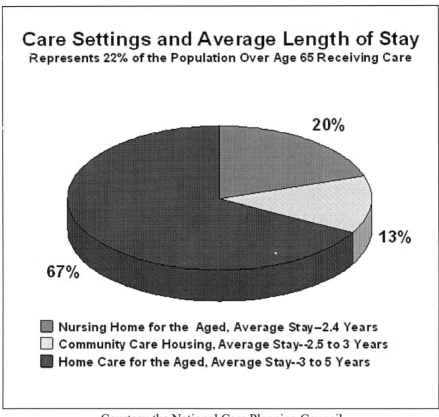

Courtesy the National Care Planning Council

Cost of Home Care

"As our society ages, the question of how we finance long term care services will become even more pressing. About 9 million adults currently receive long term care assistance, either in community settings or in nursing homes. Over 80 percent of those adults reside in the community, not in institutions. Among those 85 and older, about 55 percent require long term care assistance. Nearly 60 percent of elderly persons receiving long term care assistance rely exclusively on unpaid caregivers, primarily children and spouses. Only 7 percent of the elderly rely exclusively on paid services."
Congresswoman Nancy L. Johnson (R-CT), Chairman, Subcommittee on Health of the Committee on Ways and Means-- 2005

There is usually little ongoing cost for informal caregiving done by family members and volunteers since these services are mostly furnished free of charge. However, there is a growing trend for out-of-state or fulltime employed family caregivers to bring in paid provider services for home care. There can also be significant costs for supplies, medications, hospital equipment, and home modification even without a paid caregiver.

Supplies could include diapers, wipes, pads, and personal hygiene supplies. These are paid typically out-of-pocket and surprisingly could cost as much as $200.00 to $400.00 a month.

Hospital equipment includes such things as special air beds, walkers, wheelchairs, scooters, stools, oxygen equipment, crutches, and hospital beds. Some of this cost may be covered by Medicare, but co-pay must be made unless the recipient has a Medicare supplement policy which should pick up the additional cost.

Home modification could include building ramps, widening doorways, installing special showers and toilets, installing lifts, and handrails. These costs are borne by the care-recipient or her family.

As a general rule, government programs will not pay for any home care unless there is a medical need. Specific qualifications are necessary to receive government financial aid.

Medicare will pay for home care services on a limited basis to help a person who is homebound, recover from an injury or medical condition. Medicare provides a home health agency about 60 days worth of payment to help with the recovery. If the recipient fails to respond, deteriorates, or is not improving in any way Medicare will no longer cover the cost of care.

Local area agencies on aging, sometimes in conjunction with Medicaid, will often pay for home repairs, transportation, and snow removal for low income recipients. In addition, many low income people can receive rent subsidies and help with utility bills from Federal and local governments. The local area agency on aging can furnish information on these programs.

For people with low incomes, area agencies on aging provide some free help. There are volunteers who will sit with a care recipient to give some free time to the caregiver. There are Meals-on-Wheels at no cost or very low cost. Senior centers are usually sponsored by area agencies on aging, and they sometimes provide transportation for a disabled person at home.

The Veteran's Administration will also pay for home care for qualifying veterans on a basis similar to Medicare. Under VA rules -- as with Medicare -- there must be a medical need for care in the home. VA has additional restrictions where the recipient must have a substantial service-connected disability and must be very low income.

For people who do not qualify as low income and have assets, the cost of homecare is paid from personal funds. If the family finds it necessary to bring in a homecare agency to help with lifting, bathing, walking, incontinence, toileting, dressing, or supervision the cost could be anywhere from $12.00 to $25.00 an hour. Charges depend on the area of the country and whether there is a contract for extended weekly services.

For those who had the foresight to buy long term care insurance, the insurance will cover the cost of home care either for help with activities of daily living, with supervision for dementia, and, if it is a newer policy, for help with many of the other activities listed at the beginning of this section. These activities are called "homemaker services." Most policies will pay, in addition, for home modification and other necessary training and support to help a person remain in the home.

Adult Day Services
Other terms used for this type of care are: adult day centers, adult day care center, adult day health services, adult day residential care, and medical adult day care services.

Adult day care services have been around for about 30 years. A survey completed in 2001 put the number of adult day care centers at 3,493 nationwide. The survey by Partners in Caregiving also indicated that at least twice as many centers are needed as are currently available. The National Adult Day Services Association estimates current numbers of adult day care providers at around 4,000.

Adult day services offer an ideal alternative to caregivers by providing a daytime care environment outside of the home. The care recipient receives supervision and possibly some limited care while the caregiver has a break from the routine of daily caregiving. This gives the caregiver needed time for herself or himself and some peace and quiet to relieve the stress of caregiving. The care center might also offer transportation at an additional small cost to transport the loved one to and from the center.

There are two types of services; traditional model and health care model. The traditional model typically provides activities and supervision for older adults in a safe environment. The medical model provides nursing services, therapy, and counseling services in addition to supervision.

Housing for the Elderly Poor
According to the U.S. census bureau, in 2002, 31% of households with a member over the age of 65 made less than $1,250.00 per month. It appears from these data, roughly one in three of all elderly households are struggling to get by. For those elderly poor, who are paying rent or still paying mortgages, the census bureau estimates well over 50% of household income goes towards housing costs. It's not surprising that at least 1/3 of all housing for the poor is occupied by people over age 65. Nationwide there are 2.9 million subsidized apartments available for 5.1 million low income families that could qualify for government assistance with affordable housing. Many of these are elderly.

The elderly frequently are reluctant to find out about low income housing options and many are missing out on opportunities for comfortable housing at affordable prices. The best source for those over age 65 to find out about low income housing in their area is to contact their local area agency on aging. This is an extremely valuable resource and should be utilized. There are about 655 AAA's serving every urban and rural corner of the United States

Hospice Care

Hospice is a program involving medical personnel and volunteers to give comfort and support to someone who is expected to die within six months. Rather than trying to cure the condition causing death, hospice is designed to:

- Provide care in the home in familiar surroundings or in specially designed inpatient facilities
- Provide medication to relieve pain
- Provide appropriate physician and skilled nursing services for end-of-life care
- Provide adequate nutrition and hydration if necessary
- Give help with activities of daily living such as bathing, toileting, and feeding
- Support and give comfort to the family or family caregivers
- Provide bereavement support for the family, up to 13 months after the loved one has died

Hospice care allows terminally ill patients and their families to remain together in the comfort and dignity of the home. In addition, hospice care allows family members to take an active role in providing care or supplementing the care provided by formal caregivers such as a nurse, physician, social worker, dietitian, counselor, clergy, or volunteers. The hospice team makes regular visits and does as much caregiving as required.

Care can be provided in the home, in special hospital settings, in nursing homes, or in stand-alone hospice facilities. A lot depends on the amount of care needed.

Hospice care for the aged is a program paid for entirely by Medicare but only if the person receiving hospice is enrolled in Medicare. Fortunately, virtually everyone over age 65 is enrolled in Medicare. Medicare will not cover the cost of room and board in a facility dedicated entirely to hospice.

Community and Government
Long Term Care Programs

Government Long Term Care Programs

It is interesting to note that a large majority of the American public still believes that the government will provide long term care when needed. Care is generally only available for people with very little income and no assets. And for many services, even for these folks, there are roadblocks and waiting lists. It is this misconception about government programs that most likely prevents people from planning for care for themselves.

> **Only 16% of all long term care services are provided by the government.**

Community Groups and Services

There are many private, religious, and government organizations across the country that provide supportive services for older people. Many of these services center around helping people stay in their homes and avoid having to go to live in an institution or perhaps move in with family. Because of the emphasis on helping people remain independent, many community aging programs could be viewed as long term care programs. Community services may provide socialization or service opportunities which might include:

- Meals served at home or in community centers
- Transportation and shopping for people who can't drive
- Home repairs, yard work, telephone support, caregiver support

Private support groups in the community might include the Red Cross, United Way, women's auxiliaries or business groups. Many religious denominations support long term care services for their elderly members as well as nonmembers.

Both private and religious groups often provide services for free to people with little income and few assets. They may, however, charge people for services who have adequate income or assets. Check your phone book for local numbers for the Red Cross and United Way. Other listings may be under Community Services.

Senior Corps
Sponsored by the Corporation for National and Community Service, Senior Corps has a senior companion program where seniors 60 and older offer companionship and aid to homebound elders with visits, transportation, and friendly support. You can contact their national office or search on their website for a Senior Corps organization in your state. http://www.seniorcorps.org/

Senior Centers
Senior Centers are often the focal point for all aging services in a community. Experts or contact people are housed in senior centers and can provide information and service in the center itself or refer out to other organizations that can help. The community-served meals or congregate meals in senior centers are a means for attracting older people into the centers. Seniors can then be exposed to the many services that are available. You can locate your local senior center in your phone book under "senior centers" or "state aging services."

Administration on Aging
The Administration on Aging oversees a wide array of home and community based services for over 8 million elderly individuals each year, which is 17 percent of all people aged 60 and older - including 3 million individuals who require intensive services and meet the functional requirements for nursing home care. The agency also provides direct services to over 600,000 informal caregivers each year, who are struggling to keep their loved ones at home. This national aging network is the largest long term care provider network in the country.

There are 655 area agencies on aging in every state and territory of the United States. State aging units, under direction from the Administration on Aging, oversee and coordinate the activities of area agencies on aging in their states. Services are numerous but concentrate primarily on helping elderly people remain independent in the community, delaying the possibility that they will need help in a facility. Area agencies also support caregivers and coordinate Medicaid programs for home care and assisted living. Agencies also support caregivers and grandparents caring for their grandchildren. Here is a list of more common area agency on aging services.

- **Access Services** such as transportation, outreach, information and assistance, case management, and so on
- **In-Home Services** including homemaker and home health aides, home repair, snow removal, chore and maintenance, supportive services for families of older individuals who have Alzheimer's disease, and so on
- **Community Services** such as adult day care, senior centers, legal assistance, recreation, and so on
- **Community Served Meals** and meals on wheels

State aging departments and area agencies on aging offer limited free legal advice to qualifying persons under the Older Americans Act. The local area agency on aging has an advisory service for help with understanding Medicare, Medicare supplements, Medicare advantage, and Medicare Part D.

A local area agency on aging can be reached by dialing 211.

Eldercare Locator
1.800.677.1116
The Eldercare Locator is a national toll free referral number funded by the U.S. Administration on Aging. You can call this number with questions or needs, and they will direct you to a specialist in your area who can help you. They have information in all areas of aging services including help for caregivers. Eldercare Locator Information takes calls Monday to Friday, 9 a.m. to 8 p.m. Eastern Standard Time. Voice messaging is available 24 hours a day for you to leave a call back number.

Food Stamps
Various food and nutrition programs to help low income individuals and families are available. You must meet certain eligibility requirements. One of the most familiar programs is the Food Stamp Program. To apply to the program, you can contact your local Food Stamp office to set up an interview. You must qualify through income and asset tests.

Housing Assistance

Housing assistance programs help support and protect low income families, older Americans, and the disabled. You may seek advice from your local area agency on aging to find safer neighborhoods, low-cost housing, or services such as Meals-on-Wheels. There are government assistance housing options that include public housing, section 8 and housing choice vouchers, and section 202 housing support. The local city or county housing authority in your state, which administers housing and community development programs, is another resource for housing assistance. There are qualifying income and asset tests to qualify for housing assistance.

Low Income Energy Assistance Program

Your local Low Income Home Energy Assistance Program (LIHEAP) may be able to help you pay for your heating and/or cooling bills, or weatherization of your home. LIHEAP is a federally funded energy assistance program that is run by the nation's states and territories. You must apply for this program. Your area agency can help locate these services for you. There are qualifying income and asset tests.

Medicare

Medicare was the vision and campaign promise of President John F. Kennedy to provide universal medical insurance to all aged Americans. His untimely death did not allow him to fulfill his promise, but President Lyndon Johnson was able to win passage of the plan in the form of amendments to the Social Security Act. Passed in 1965, Title VIII of the amendment established Medicare and Title IX established Medicaid.

Medicare Part A and B is now the health insurance plan for all eligible individuals age 65 and older and certain younger disabled persons. Medicare Part D is the drug prescription program. (*More detail about Medicare payments for long term care under STEP 2)*

Medicaid

Medicaid is an assistance program for certain low income people. These include: low income families with children; people age 65 or older meeting asset and income tests, blind or disabled people on Supplemental Security Income; certain low income pregnant women and their children, certain types of cancer patients, and people who have very high medical bills and qualify financially.

Medicaid is funded by the Federal Government with matching funds from the States. It is largely administered through each individual state. Although there are broad federal requirements for Medicaid, states have a wide degree of flexibility to design their programs. States have authority to establish eligibility standards, determine what benefits and services to cover, and set payment rates. Eligibility and services thus vary in each state. All states, however, must cover these basic services:

- inpatient and outpatient hospital services
- laboratory and X-ray services
- skilled nursing home care
- home health services
- doctor's services
- family planning
- diagnosis and treatment for children

Medicaid is for young people and old people alike. State spending for old people for long term care services has been increasing at an accelerating rate. Nationwide about 35% of all Medicaid expenditures are for long term care services for the elderly.

Eligibility requirements for Medicaid long term care can vary for each state, but all states require adult age to be 65 unless mentally retarded, developmentally disabled or blind. Also income and asset eligibility for the state must be met. Because each state sets its own rules, you could qualify in one state and not in another. (*More detail about Medicaid requirements and funds under STEP 2*)

Veterans Affairs Long Term Care Services
The US Department of Veterans Affairs provides three types of long term care services for veterans.

The first are benefits provided to veterans who have service-connected disabilities. These services include home care, assisted living -- or as it is sometimes called, domiciliary care -- and nursing home care. There are strict income and service-connected disability requirements for receiving this care.

The second benefit is state veterans homes. VA, in conjunction with the states, helps build and support state veterans homes. Money is provided to help with construction and a daily subsidy is provided each veteran using these homes. The majority of these facilities offer nursing care, but some may also offer assisted living, domiciliary and even adult day care. These homes are generally available for any veteran regardless of status and are run by the states, often with the help of contract management. Many states have waiting lists.

The third benefit for veterans is the "aid and attendance benefit" under the Improved Pension or Death Pension. All active-duty veterans who served during a period of war are eligible for the pension and the aid and attendance or housebound allowance. Their surviving spouse and dependent children are also eligible for a lesser amount of death pension benefit and allowances Veterans under the age of 65 must be totally disabled; however, veterans age 65 and over, regardless of health, are considered totally disabled due to age and there is no requirement to prove disability.

This can be an extremely helpful benefit for paying the costs of home care, assisted living or nursing homes. There are income and asset tests to qualify for this benefit.

(More detail about Long Term Care Benefits for Veterans under STEP 2)

STEP 2

Funding the Costs of Long Term Care

Having funds to pay for care expands
the choices for care settings and providers.

Determining the Cost of Long Term Care

In order to plan financially for long term care, you need to know what the costs are now and what they will be in the future.

Every year MetLife conducts a national survey of nursing home, assisted living, and home health agency costs. This is a valuable resource for determining the cost of care in your area. You can view the September 2007 results on their website. Type "MetLife nursing home survey" in a Google search. MetLife also publishes a survey on assisted living and home care costs. The search above should give you access to those data as well.

According to MetLife's 2007 survey the National average cost of a nursing home, private room is $213 per day, $77,745 annually. Cost of semi-private room is $189 per day, $68,985 annually. Home care aide average cost is $19 per hour.

Taking into account the cost of long term care today with added inflation to future costs, it makes sense to take steps now to secure finances.

We know that government programs such as Medicare, Medicaid, and Veterans Affairs will cover the cost of long term care under certain conditions. Medicare will cover rehabilitation from a hospital stay or limited care at home if there is a skilled medical need. However, when the skilled medical need ends, so does Medicare payment.

Medicaid will cover both medical and non-medical related long term care, but in order to qualify for Medicaid, a person has to have less than $2,000 in assets and income that is insufficient to pay the cost of care. In other words a person must be impoverished.

The VA hospitals will provide nursing home care and provide home care services for those who served in the military, but due to lack of funding and strict qualification rules not many veterans qualify for this care.

Before you use any of these government resources, you will probably find yourself paying out-of-pocket expenses for informal home care and facing financial decisions that will erode your hard-won assets. Financial preparation done years in advance eliminates a large part of the stress that goes with long term care. It is well-documented that caregiving stress causes illness, aging related problems, and often a premature death for the caregiver.

Savings or Asset Conversions to Pay for Long Term Care

Contingency Funding

A contingency fund is money set aside in cash or investments that can easily and quickly be liquidated to pay for long term care. The fund can take two forms: 1) monthly cash payments set aside over a long period or 2) retirement savings that are not spent or that are being hoarded in old age.

As a rule, if a person can't qualify for long term care insurance, then setting aside money is the next best alternate. However, if buying insurance is an option, then it is much cheaper than a set-aside. Depending on when care is needed, the set-aside can cost anywhere from 5 times to 20,000 times the cost of insurance premiums.

You Need to Know How Much to Put Away

The chart below will help you determine how much money you have to put away monthly in order to fund the future cost of long term care services.

The form also assumes that the cost of care increases by 5% per year. This means that 14 years from now the same service costing $5,000 today will cost $10,000.

Now let's use the table. We are using the current table assumptions of $5,000 a month of costs increasing annually by 5%. Suppose you want to know how much money to put away every month from now until 20 years from now when you will need care. Go down the column labeled "years" to the number 20. In the columns to the right determine how many years of care you want. For example, 5 years of care 20 years from now would require $758,085 (Future dollars). Now go to the shaded columns on the far right and find the corresponding 5 year benefit column. Go down that column to the 20th year and the amount in the box is the monthly amount you need to set aside for the next 20 years to fund 5 years worth of care. This amount is $1,881 per month.

Determining The Amount of Money to Set Aside For Care

Monthly payments needed to fund $5000 a month in
care costs @ 5% earnings, a 5% annual increase in costs
and adjusted for a 25% Federal and state income tax rate.

Monthly Long Term Care Cost -- $5,000
Current State and Federal Income Tax -- 25.0%
Yearly Increase in Long Term Care Cost -- 5.0%
Earnings Adjusted for Taxes -- 5.0%

Years	Date	1 Year's Worth of Future Benefit Costs	2 Years' Worth of Future Benefit Costs	3 Years' Worth of Future Benefit Costs	5 Years' Worth of Future Benefit Costs	Monthly Payment for a 1 Year Benefit	Monthly Payment for a 2 Year Benefit	Monthly Payment for a 3 Year Benefit	Monthly Payment for a 5 Year Benefit
1	2007	$60,000	$120,000	$180,000	$300,000	$4,984	$9,968	$14,953	$24,921
2	2008	$63,000	$126,000	$189,000	$315,000	$2,551	$5,103	$7,654	$12,757
3	2009	$66,150	$132,300	$198,450	$330,750	$1,741	$3,482	$5,223	$8,705
4	2010	$69,458	$138,915	$208,373	$347,288	$1,336	$2,673	$4,009	$6,682
5	2011	$72,930	$145,861	$218,791	$364,652	$1,094	$2,188	$3,282	$5,469
6	2012	$76,577	$153,154	$229,731	$382,884	$932	$1,865	$2,797	$4,662
7	2013	$80,406	$160,811	$241,217	$402,029	$817	$1,635	$2,452	$4,087
8	2014	$84,426	$168,852	$253,278	$422,130	$731	$1,463	$2,194	$3,657
9	2015	$88,647	$177,295	$265,942	$443,237	$665	$1,329	$1,994	$3,323
10	2016	$93,080	$186,159	$279,239	$465,398	$611	$1,223	$1,834	$3,057
11	2017	$97,734	$195,467	$293,201	$488,668	$568	$1,136	$1,704	$2,840
12	2018	$102,620	$205,241	$307,861	$513,102	$532	$1,064	$1,596	$2,660
13	2019	$107,751	$215,503	$323,254	$538,757	$502	$1,003	$1,505	$2,508
14	2020	$113,139	$226,278	$339,417	$565,695	$476	$951	$1,427	$2,378
15	2021	$118,796	$237,592	$356,388	$593,979	$453	$907	$1,360	$2,267
16	2022	$124,736	$249,471	$374,207	$623,678	$434	$868	$1,302	$2,169
17	2023	$130,972	$261,945	$392,917	$654,862	$417	$834	$1,250	$2,084
18	2024	$137,521	$275,042	$412,563	$687,605	$402	$803	$1,205	$2,008
19	2025	$144,397	$288,794	$433,191	$721,986	$388	$777	$1,165	$1,941
20	2026	$151,617	$303,234	$454,851	$758,085	$376	$752	$1,129	$1,881
21	2027	$159,198	$318,396	$477,594	$795,989	$365	$731	$1,096	$1,827
22	2028	$167,158	$334,316	$501,473	$835,789	$356	$711	$1,067	$1,778
23	2029	$175,516	$351,031	$526,547	$877,578	$347	$694	$1,041	$1,734
24	2030	$184,291	$368,583	$552,874	$921,457	$339	$678	$1,016	$1,694
25	2031	$193,506	$387,012	$580,518	$967,530	$331	$663	$994	$1,657
26	2032	$203,181	$406,363	$609,544	$1,015,906	$325	$649	$974	$1,624
27	2033	$213,340	$426,681	$640,021	$1,066,702	$319	$637	$956	$1,593
28	2034	$224,007	$448,015	$672,022	$1,120,037	$313	$626	$938	$1,564
29	2035	$235,208	$470,415	$705,623	$1,176,039	$308	$615	$923	$1,538
30	2036	$246,968	$493,936	$740,904	$1,234,841	$303	$605	$908	$1,513

Sale of Assets

Tangible assets that might produce enough income to pay for long term care might include investment property such as rentals, commercially leased property, land, a farm, second home, or a business.

Some individuals are heavy into real estate and short on cash. If the intent was to cash out of the investment at some future point, then a sale is warranted. However, it seems a shame to sacrifice in early years to establish an investment only to throw it away to long term care. It would make more sense to use income from the investments to buy long term care insurance.

Sale of a Home You Are Living in to Pay for Long Term Care

Selling the home can give you cash needed to pay for assisted living facility, or if you are going to live with children, it would give money for home care services.

There are real estate specialists called Seniors Real Estate Specialists (SRES) who are trained especially for senior sales and moves. If it is urgent that the sale and move be made, they are the ones to contact. They handle every aspect of the move to even settling you into your new living quarters. You can read more about SRES and locate a specialist in your area on www.longtermcarelink.net.

Reverse Mortgage

A reverse mortgage is a special type of loan used by older Americans to convert the equity in their homes into cash. The money obtained through a reverse mortgage can provide seniors with the financial security they need to fully enjoy their retirement years.

The reverse mortgage is aptly named because the payment stream is reversed. Instead of the borrower making monthly payments to a lender, as with a regular first mortgage or home equity loan, a lender makes payments to the borrower. While a reverse mortgage loan is outstanding, the borrower owns the home (just like any other mortgage) and holds title to it but does not make any monthly mortgage payments.

The loan becomes due and payable when the borrower ceases to occupy their home as a principal residence. This can occur if the survivor (the last remaining spouse, in cases of couples) passes away, sells the home, or permanently moves out of the home. The home does not have to be sold to pay off the loan. The borrower, or the borrower's heirs, can instead pay off the reverse mortgage and keep the home.

The money from a reverse mortgage can be used for ANYTHING: daily living expenses, home repairs and home improvements, medical bills and prescription drugs, payoff of existing debts, education, travel, long term health care, prevention of foreclosure, and other needs. In fact, by paying off debt or an existing mortgage, the reverse mortgage can allow you to stay in your home and receive care.

The size of the reverse mortgage that you can get will depends on your age -- or ages if a couple -- at the time you apply for the loan, the type of reverse mortgage you choose, the value of your home, current interest rates, and where you live. In general, the older you are and the more valuable your home -- and the less you owe on your home --, the larger the reverse mortgage can be. The cash from the reverse mortgage can be paid to you by:

1. A single lump sum of cash
2. A regular monthly cash advance
3. A line of credit account from which you take cash as needed (The line of credit balance also earns interest which allows this account to grow.)

There are some costs to originating the loan, such as appraisal fees, mortgage insurance and other charges similar to regular mortgage loans. All of these fees can be rolled into the loan resulting in no out-of-pocket costs for doing a reverse mortgage.

The money provided to you from a reverse mortgage is tax-free; it is not income that you must pay taxes on. However, the funds received from a reverse mortgage may affect your eligibility for certain kinds of government assistance. You should check this before getting a reverse mortgage.

We recommend you use a reverse mortgage specialist. You can read more about reverse mortgages and locate a specialist in your area on www.longtermcarelink.net.

Long Term Care Insurance

Why buy long term care insurance

1. It will help you keep your independence and dignity and allow you to make choices. When the time comes for paying for your long term care needs, you may end up spending your savings and then relying on Medicaid for assistance. Medicaid typically pays for a semi-private room in a nursing home, but not all nursing homes take Medicaid. In many states it is not easy to get Medicaid to cover home care or pay for assisted living. Many people want to stay at home, but with Medicaid may not be able to. <u>Insurance allows you to have a choice of where you want to live.</u>

2. If you are married and you have a need for long term care, your spouse may be forced to pay for an outside caregiver. The cost is likely to come from your combined income and assets. This may leave your spouse with minimal funds in the future. <u>Insurance solves this problem and allows the healthy spouse to keep the assets.</u>

3. Many healthy caregiving spouses won't spend their money and choose to "tough it out" on their own without help. If care of a disabled spouse drags on too long, this can have a devastating effect on the physical and emotion health of the caregiver. <u>Insurance will pay for professional care for the disabled spouse and allow the caregiver spouse needed rest.</u>

4. If your children promise to take care of you when the time comes that you need care, insurance will help them do that. Probably neither you nor your children have thought of the prospects of moving you from place to place, changing your dirty diapers, cleaning up after "accidents" in the bathroom or helping you with bathing and dressing. <u>Insurance will pay for aides to help your children with these tasks.</u>

5. If you are single and a need for long term care arises, insurance can pay for and coordinate that care. <u>With insurance you won't have to feel you would be a burden for family or friends.</u>

6. <u>If you have the desire to leave assets behind when you die, insurance will help preserve those assets from the cost of long term care.</u>

Buy Long Term Care Insurance When You Are Younger

There is a bonus to buying long term care insurance at a younger age. The yearly premium is lower and the total premium over the life of the policy is also less. For example, a person in good health, currently age 45, buying a typical policy with inflation protection, could spend $42,075 in total premiums to age 78. The yearly premium for this policy is $1,275.

Suppose this same person chooses to wait to buy the equivalent coverage-- adjusted for inflation -- at age 65. If that same policy were available in the future, he could pay $44,759 in total premiums over his 13 remaining years to age 78. His premium is also considerably higher and in this case is $3,443 a year. By waiting, he saves no money in total cost, he will have a much higher yearly cost and in addition will definitely incur the following risks:

- The same policies only stick around about three years and historically, new policies invariably have higher rates for the same ages as older ones. This means, all else being equal, he could pay two or three times more in total cost for an equivalent policy in the future.
- The policy at age 45 is based on the best health rating and someone age 65 is very unlikely to get that same rating which means a much more expensive total cost in the future.
- By waiting, his health may deteriorate to a point where he can't even qualify for a policy. Unfortunately, we have seen this happen time and time again to people who wait and all of a sudden desperately want coverage because of a change in health and can't get it.
- He may need long term care before he turns 65. The chances of incurring a disability prior to age 65 are quite high.
- We recommend you work with a long term care insurance specialist who understands the policy provisions and the coverage needed and can help you determine the best policy for what you want.

How to buy long term care insurance

Here is a checklist of some of the things you need to know before you purchase a policy.

LONG TERM CARE INSURANCE BUYING CHECKLIST
the more "yes" answers you get the better off you are.

1) Is the insurance company rated by A. M. Best (the rating company) with a rating of at least A, A+ or A++?

2) Is it a large diversified company with deep pockets and selling more than just long term care insurance?

3) Is the insurance representative an expert in long term care insurance? (Because of its complexity, almost all LTCi experts only sell LTCi; they seldom sell anything else.)

4) Does the representative have a degree and/or industry financial designations?

5) Does the representative own a personal long term care insurance policy for himself or herself?

6) Is the policy you like tax qualified, and if not, do you understand the ramifications?

7) Are there at least 6 ADL's (Activities of Daily Living) allowed for in the benefit certification?

8) Does it allow "standby assistance"?

9) Is it a "pool of money" as opposed to a "stated period"?

10) Is it "integrated" as opposed to "2-pool"? (2-pool is not allowed in some states.)

11) Do you understand how the elimination period works? (This is extremely important.)

12) Does it have prohibitive cost containment provisions?

13) Is there any "capping" of automatic benefit increase riders?

14) Do you understand how the waiver of premium works?

15) Does the assisted living facility benefit pay the same as for nursing home?

16) Are you buying adequate home care coverage?

17) Does the company have a history of premium rate stability without periodic increases?

18) Does the policy pay for homemaker services?

19) Does the policy offer an alternative plan of care for services that don't exist today?

Using Life insurance to Create Extra Income

Getting Money Out of Life Insurance without Dying

- Borrow against the cash value of the life insurance policy.
- Instruct the life insurance carrier to cash out the policy, based on the available cash surrender value.
- Determine if the life insurance carrier offers an "accelerated benefits program" rider and if the insured is eligible.
- Sell the life insurance policy in a life settlement.
- Borrow from friends or family using the life insurance policy as collateral to secure the loan.
- A combination of an "accelerated benefit" and a life settlement may be possible and might net more cash than either by itself!

We recommend checking with your life insurance agent or company on determining availability to obtain money from your policy and if this serves your best interests.

Life Settlements

In recent years, a large and growing industry has emerged where major investment groups, mutual funds or hedge funds purchase the life insurance policies owned by older Americans. The purchasers become the new owners and beneficiaries for the death benefits of these purchased policies. They also take over paying the premiums. This is a legitimate investment in the death of another person. The investor will pay the insured 20% to 80% of the face value of the policy depending on the age and health of the seller.

Policies generally have to have a face value of more than $100,000 and in order to receive a reasonable purchase price for the policy; the owner should not be expected to live much longer than three to five years. For those life insurance owners who also need long term care, this is an excellent way to free up money to pay for the immediate costs of that care.

You can read more about life settlements and locate a specialist in your area on www.longtermcarelink.net.

Annuities

Income Annuities (Converting Assets to Income)

Income annuities are often a good strategy for seniors who are concerned about outliving their assets. The mindset of most seniors is to hold onto cash and not give it up. On the other hand, a senior could convert cash into income in the form of a guaranteed single premium income annuity. A guaranteed income stream for someone who is likely to live a long time is a good retirement planning strategy. This does not mean that all cash needs to be converted into income. A good strategy is to find a balance and retain some cash and convert some to income.

Converting assets to income is also often a good strategy to preserve assets from Medicaid spend down and to qualify for veterans "aid and attendance." Setting up an income stream many years in advance of the need for Medicaid will also allow for income options that Medicaid would not allow were the income annuity purchased for Medicaid planning during the spend down process.

Deferred Annuities

Many seniors purchase single premium deferred annuities for a stable interest rate on their savings or to defer payment of income taxes on the earnings.

One disadvantage of deferred annuities is unfavorable tax treatment for estate planning purposes. If the deferred annuity is being purchased to pass money on to the next generation, there are better options. If the deferred annuity is being purchased for future consumption by the owner, then estate planning should not be an issue.

For those who have purchased a deferred annuity and would like to fix the unfavorable estate planning features, there is a potential correction for that. If the senior or the senior couple is relatively healthy, proceeds from the annuity can be used to purchase single or joint life insurance with a death benefit equal to the value of the annuity. Life insurance proceeds pass to named beneficiaries of the next generation without taxes. Thus the value of the annuity can be transferred tax free.

Some sources make a claim that money in a deferred annuity is not subject to Medicaid asset qualification rules. This is not true. This claim is actually based on the idea of putting money into the deferred annuity and then triggering the income option inside the annuity, converting it to an income stream and using it as a Medicaid annuity. This is legitimate but the annuity agent often forgets to mention this as part of the strategy.

If a senior understands the strategy above and is satisfied with it as a Medicaid planning tool, then tying up money in this manner may be an acceptable option. If a senior does not understand the strategy and is being induced to buy an annuity based on a false claim, there is no reason to tie up money in a deferred annuity to create a Medicaid income annuity. The Medicaid annuity can be purchased at any time with funds held in any type of account. The funds do not have to be held inside a deferred annuity.

Medicaid Annuities
Medicaid annuities work by converting assets, that would normally be spent down to qualify for Medicaid, into income that can be used by the healthy spouse. By converting those spend down assets into income, the Medicaid beneficiary accelerates his or her qualification for Medicaid benefits.

This technique works in most states as long as the annuity is set up using Medicaid guidelines and it is irrevocable. New rules from the deficit reduction act of 2006 require that these annuities name the state Medicaid as a beneficiary if the annuity has a remainder benefit at the death of the owner. Medicaid annuities are used primarily to convert assets into income for a healthy spouse not receiving Medicaid. The purpose is to provide a larger income for this so-called community spouse than would be available under normal Medicaid rules.

Here are the government guidelines for Medicaid annuities from HCFA Transmittal 64:

"When an individual purchases an annuity, he or she generally pays to the entity issuing the annuity (e.g., a bank or insurance company) a lump sum of money, in return for which he or she is promised regular payments of income in certain amounts. These payments may continue for a fixed period of time (for example, 10 years) or for as long as the individual (or another designated beneficiary) lives, thus creating an ongoing income stream. Annuities, although usually purchased in order to provide a source of income for retirement, are occasionally used to shelter assets so that individuals purchasing them can become eligible for Medicaid. In order to avoid penalizing annuities validly purchased as part of a retirement plan but to capture those annuities".

"The average number of years of expected life remaining for the individual must coincide with the life of the annuity. If the individual is not reasonably expected to live longer than the guarantee period of the annuity, the individual will not receive fair market value for the annuity based on the projected return. In this case, the annuity is not actuarially sound and a transfer of assets for less than fair market value has taken place, subjecting the individual to a penalty. The penalty is assessed based on a transfer of assets for less than fair market value that is considered to have occurred at the time the annuity was purchased".

"For example, if a male at age 65 purchases a $10,000 annuity to be paid over the course of 10 years, his life expectancy according to the table is 14.96 years. Thus, the annuity is actuarially sound. However, if a male at age 80 purchases the same annuity for $10,000 to be paid over the course of 10 years, his life expectancy is only 6.98 years. Thus, a payout of the annuity for approximately 3 years is considered a transfer of assets for less than fair market value and that amount is subject to penalty."

If the Medicaid annuity fits your planning situation, you need to do it right and you need to follow the rules in your particular state regarding Medicaid annuities.

We recommend you talk to a qualified elder law attorney to help you with Medicaid annuities. You can read more about annuity products and locate a specialist in your area on www.longtermcarelink.net

Government Programs That Pay for Long Term Care

Medicare Long Term Care Coverage

Medicare Part A -- Inpatient Hospital (2008)
Medicare pays hospital care with deductibles as outlined here. You pay the deductible or if you purchase medicare supplemental insurance it will pay the deductible.

- $1,024 Deductible - First 60 Days
- $256/Day Coinsurance - 61st Through 90th Day
- $512/Day Coinsurance - 91st Through 150th Day
- Beyond 150 Days You Or Your Supplement Insurance Pay The Total Cost
- There Is A One Time, "Lifetime Reserve" Of 60 Days That Medicare Will Also Pay.

Under Part A, you are also allowed 3 pints of blood.

Medicare Skilled Nursing Facility -- Nursing Home (2008)
To qualify for medicare nursing home coverage, you must spend at least three full days in a hospital and must have a skilled nursing need and have a doctor order it. The transfer from a hospital must occur within a certain time period. Medicare may pay up to 100 days for a stay in a nursing home. This depends on the medical need. There is a coinsurance payment after the 20th day. Most Medicare supplement insurance will pick up this out-of-pocket amount.

- $0 deductible for the first 20 days
- $128/day coinsurance - 21st through 100th day
- After the 100th day or possibly even before that time, if a skilled nursing need or other qualifications are not met, medicare will stop paying. At this time the medicare supplement insurance stops paying also. You will be responsible for all costs after this point unless you have long term care insurance. Long term care insurance will begin to pay after medicare stops.

Medicare will not pay nursing home costs for someone admitted from his or her home. Almost half of those admitted to nursing care come directly from home.

Medicare Part A (Also Part B) -- Home Health Care
To qualify for Medicare home care coverage, a person must be under a "plan of care" by a doctor. There must be a skilled need requiring frequent visits. Those skilled services might include:

- Nursing services by RN or LPN
- Physical therapy
- Social services
- Homemaker services
- Occupational therapy
- Physician services
- Speech therapy
- Nutrition services

Medicare home care is often used for covering patients who are recovering from hip surgery, foot surgery, joint replacement, or complications of diabetes. At times, congestive heart failure or other disabling conditions require home care. When skilled care is not needed, Medicare stops.

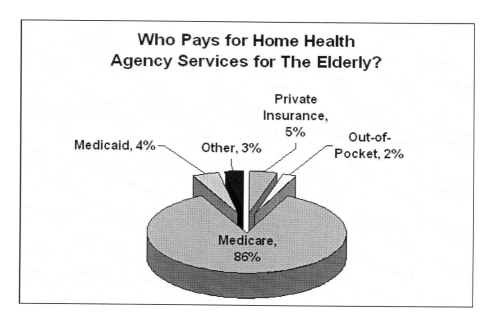

Source: 2005 statistical abstract of the United States

Medicare pays for about 86% of all home care that meets the criteria of skilled home care services. Companies that provide these services are called "home health agencies."

Medicare Hospice
When death is expected within six months or health is deteriorating quickly overturned as, hospice care prescribed by a physician is 100% covered by Medicare.

Medicare Part B
Medicare Part B covers outpatient services and doctors. This is an optional plan from Medicare to help pay for outpatient and doctors care. This plan must be signed up for during your enrollment period. There is a monthly premium which is deducted from your Social Security payment. The amount does increase each year. In 2005 it was $78.20 per month. There is also an annual deductible. Part B premiums and deductibles go up every year. Medicare Supplement Insurance usually pays for deductibles and co-pays not covered by Medicare.

- Monthly payment for Medicare Part B -- $96.40 per month in 2008
- Annual deductible - $135 per calendar year in 2008
- Medicare pays 80% of most services, leaving 20% paid by coinsurance or personal funds
- Certain lab tests and vaccines are paid at 100%

Medicare part B may also cover certain durable medical equipment for home care such as hospital bed, walker, etc.

- $0 deductible - Home health Care under physicians prescription for skilled need is paid 100%
- $135 deductible and 20% coinsurance for "Durable Medical Equipment"

Medicare Supplement Insurance
Medicare supplement insurance or Medi-Gap plans are not government insurance policies. There are many private insurance companies that sell medicare supplement policies. These policies are designed specifically to cover the deductible and co-pay amounts

not covered by Medicare. They do not cover any other insurance needs. When Medicare stops paying, this policy also stops paying. As of 2006 they can offer no prescription drug coverage.

Medicare Part D, Prescription Drug Plans
The plan design for the new Prescription Drug Plan (PDP) is outlined in the Medicare modernization act of 2003. It includes the following features for 2008:

- The first $275 of drug costs per year must be paid by the insured, 100% out-of-pocket as a yearly deductible
- The next $2,510 in drug costs are covered 25% by the insured and 75% by the plan. (Total drug costs now equal $3,216 and total out-of-pocket now equals $834 not including monthly premiums) At this point the plan has paid 67% of drug costs and the insured has paid 33%.
- The next $2,516 of drug costs must be paid 100% by the insured, the plan pays nothing. (Total drug costs now equal $5,726 and total out-of-pocket now equals $4,050 not including monthly premiums.) At this point coverage has regressed and the plan has only paid 29% of total drug costs and the insured has paid 71% of total drug costs. This bizarre lapse in coverage feature in the plan is called the "coverage gap" or more commonly referred to as the "doughnut hole." Unlike normal insurance ,where as costs go up, and the insurance picks up an ever increasing portion of the tab, this insurance goes backwards for a portion of expenses and the insured picks up an ever increasing portion of the tab. After getting past this lapse in coverage, the insurance again picks up the cost.
- All drug costs after $5,726 or $4,050 out of pocket are paid at 5% of cost by the insured and 95% of cost by the plan.
- Spending thresholds and out-of-pocket amounts will increase each year adjusted by inflation. All of the amounts above increase each year with inflation.

PDP insurance plans can only be sold by private companies or regional Blue Cross plans that have presented bids to Medicare and have been accepted and approved to sell these plans in various regions in the country. The plans can be sold as stand alone drug coverage or they can be included in Medicare PPO and HMO

Advantage Plans. Drug plans sold in conjunction with private Fee for Service Advantage Plans are considered stand alone plans.

These plans cannot be sold through Medigap or supplemental insurance policies. Existing HMO Medicare private plans not offering drug plans will be adding these plans and private HMOs already offering drug coverage may modify their coverage to include a new PDP. Employers who offer drug coverage to retired employees are allowed to offer these plans as a replacement for existing coverage. The plan provider for employee plans will likely be one or more of the insurance companies allowed to sell this insurance by Medicare.

Medicare Advantage Plans
Over 300 private insurance companies provide Advantage Plans funded by Medicare but designed and administered by the private companies. Plans look less like traditional Medicare and more like modern group insurance. Most of these plans also incorporate the new Medicare prescription drug coverage. Medicare Advantage along with the new Medicare drug plan was created by the Medicare Modernization Act of 2003.

Congress' intent in introducing new Advantage Plans was to modernize Medicare coverage and make it look like existing catastrophic plans; but, at the same time provide lower out-of-pocket cost for traditional Medicare beneficiaries who are buying Medicare supplement policies. The Advantage Plan, for a lower premium, or perhaps no premium at all, would replace the more expensive combination of traditional Medicare and supplement plans.

Seniors who are not healthy are probably better off under traditional Medicare with the supplement insurance plan. This is because they are paying the costs of 100% coverage spread out, at a fixed cost, on a monthly basis through supplement premiums. This is contrasted with a $1,500 to $3,000 one-time, out-of-pocket co-pay per year for receiving services through an Advantage Plan. Some seniors just don't have very large sums of money in their savings and prepaying care through monthly premiums for Medicare supplement is a way to buy expensive health services on an installment plan.

Advantage Plans generally cover nursing home care differently from traditional Medicare. Traditional Medicare pays the first 20 days of nursing home services free of charge and the next 80 days of care requires a co-payment. On the other hand, most advantage plans require an up front co-payment and then will cover the nursing home at 100% thereafter.

Home care services are also covered differently. Traditional Medicare will provide funding for up to 60 days of care. Most Advantage plans will only approve care on a day to day basis. Evidence is mounting that these plans only cover about 20% of the home care normally covered by traditional Medicare.

Medicaid Long Term Care (Medi-Cal in California)

Income and Asset Eligibility Requirements
Medicaid (Medi-Cal) requires an asset (resource) and income test for qualification. You cannot qualify unless all assets are less than $2,000. For a couple applying together it is $3,000.

This asset test includes all investment properties owned, savings accounts and personal-owned assets in excess of $500, such as recreational vehicles, antique furniture, paintings, jewelry, etc. For a couple, all assets are considered jointly owned regardless of individual ownership. In some states, IRAs and 401(k)s and other tax qualified savings accounts, owned by the spouse not needing Medicaid, are excluded. In most states, assets belonging to a qualified savings account (IRA, 401(k), 403(b) etc.) by someone older than age 70 1/2 are usually considered income due to the mandatory withdrawal requirements. These assets would be excluded from the asset test.

Certain other assets are excluded and do not stand in the way of qualifying for Medicaid (Medi-Cal). Some of these may be:

- A home if you live in it, expect to return to it, or be spouse lives in it.
- The cash value of life insurance under $1,500.
- A family business if needed to sustain family members.
- Tools or trade property if needed for support of family.
- The value of burial plot.

- A funeral plan.
- An automobile if needed by the spouse or for making income
- Wedding rings and household effects

With most states there is not an income threshold test for Medicaid long term care. In those states, if income is insufficient to pay for care, then Medicaid makes up the difference. This income test is called "medically needy."

A growing number of states will not pay for Medicaid long term care if a person makes more than 300% of SSI. SSI is a welfare payment from Social Security. In 2008, 300% of SSI is equivalent to a monthly income of $1,910. Federal law requires states with an income test to allow a potential beneficiary to place income and assets in a "Miller Trust" in order to qualify if income is too high.

If a person has to pay for long term care out-of-pocket, and his or her income cannot cover that total cost, Medicaid will cover the balance. There are income and asset protection rules for couples so that the healthy spouse can take back some of the income and assets from the person needing nursing home care for living expenses.

Medicaid (Medi-Cal) Nursing Home Qualifications
You will most likely never require Medicaid assistance until there is a nursing home need. Note that in some states Medicaid will also pay for home care services and assisted living care, but the criterion for care might still based on the need for nursing home services. At that time you will apply for Medicaid. On the application you will be required to list all your income and assets. If you are married, your spouse will also need to list her or his income and assets. There are different requirements for each state, and Medicaid rules can be complicated.

Seek an Expert on Medicaid to Help You through This Process.
There are asset protection rules that allow a minimum amount of assets to be retained by the healthy spouse to avoid impoverishment. Each state sets its own limit. In 2008, the healthy spouse keeps a minimum of $20,880 dollars. In some states the minimum amount the healthy spouse can keep is more than the $20,880. Federal rules will not allow the healthy spouse to keep more than $104,800 of the combined assets. Medicaid rules allow for hardship hearings and

oftentimes such a hearing will allow the healthy spouse to keep more than $104,800. Here are some examples of the asset division rules.

1. Couple has $210,000 in combined assets. For her husband to qualify for Medicaid, the assets are divided creating $105,000 for each. Medicaid rules state that the healthy spouse can only have $104,800. The balance is assigned to the husband and has to be spent down to less than $2,000 before the husband becomes eligible for Medicaid assistance.

2. Couple has $35,000 in assets. When husband enters the nursing home, the assets are divided creating $17,500 for each. The particular state in which they live allows the spouse to keep $25,000 to avoid impoverishment. We disregard the division amount and only $10,000 must be spent down to less than $2,000 for the husband to qualify for Medicaid.

The minimum and maximum asset amounts are called by Medicaid "resource standards," and these amounts go up every year with inflation.

Unlike assets, income does not have to be shared. In some cases, this may cause impoverishment of the healthy spouse. As an example, suppose the couple has $4,000 of income but $3,000 of it belongs to the person in the nursing home, and according to Medicaid rules, must be spent on nursing home care. This leaves the healthy spouse at home with only $1,000 of income. Medicaid recognizes this may cause a hardship and allows monies from the Medicaid spouse to be added to the healthy spouse's income to bring that income up to at least $1,711.25 a month. (2008 amount)

Some states may set this level higher, but the federal rules state that, with the give back, the spouse's income cannot total more than $2,610 a month. The exception to this would be, of course, if the spouse actually personally owns more than $2,610 a month in income. These federal minimum and maximum income allowances go up each year with inflation.

Medicaid (Medi-Cal) Spend Down Strategies

Most people going through the Medicaid asset spend down process, in order to receive Medicaid benefits, don't know that the money can be spent on anything -- not just care. Money does have to be spent on behalf of the person applying for Medicaid. As an example, if the applicant has $50,000, $10,000 of that could be set aside to cover two or three months worth of nursing home costs and the other $40,000 could be spent for something else. The set aside is necessary since it may take two or three months to get the Medicaid application approved in preparation for qualification.

Perhaps the money could be put into repairing the home or buying a new car (an exempt asset) for the spouse or a myriad of other purchases. Or perhaps, the Medicaid beneficiary could hire one of his children to take care of him. If done properly, this is perfectly legal.

You should consult an elder law attorney about possible spend down strategies since putting money into the wrong purchase could disqualify a person for Medicaid.

Medicaid (Medi-Cal) Level of Care Eligibility for Nursing Homes

An individual must go through an evaluation with a state Medicaid worker in order to determine a need for care. Sometimes nursing homes are also authorized to do this evaluation. If the individual fails to meet the minimum level of care needed to qualify for that state's Medicaid coverage, then no Medicaid help is forthcoming.

A person might meet the Medicaid need for care criteria from one state but not those of another state. At times families will consider moving loved ones who have been declined in one state, to live with a member of the family in another state and possibly get qualification in that state.

Younger mentally ill, retarded, and developmentally disabled people are typically provided services in special Medicaid intermediate care facilities licensed for this type of care or in special homes maintained by the state. Remember, about 46% of all people receiving long term care are under the age of 65. These younger people are typically those just mentioned, and most of them are probably receiving Medicaid help.

Medicaid (Medi-Cal) Estate Recovery

Federal legislation in 1993 made it mandatory for states to attempt to recover Medicaid payments made on behalf of recipients from their estates after they die. Since most tangible assets are spent through Medicaid spend down, estate recovery focuses on real property, personal property, or business ownership that the deceased had an interest in prior to receiving Medicaid.

Recovery applies to individuals who were age 55 or older when they received Medicaid or to permanently institutionalized adults under 55. In a few states, recovery can also occur from the estate of living recipients who are in a nursing home and who have been certified that they cannot reasonably be expected to be discharged and return home. If it is a house, as an example, Medicaid can place a lien on the property. Most states allow a single recipient to keep the house and don't place a lien until after the death. Some states forgive the debt entirely if the surviving spouse is still living in the home.

Federal law actually allows states to file a "TEFRA Lien" against real properties while the Medicaid recipient is alive. This prevents the family from selling the property at the death of the recipient until the lien is satisfied. Not all states use this method. They rely instead on the probate process to establish a claim and a lien against property. In these states, property in a trust will sometimes evade the recovery process.

If a person had a spouse living in the home at the time of Medicaid qualification, the home did not have to be counted as a resource for the qualifying beneficiary. Yet at the death or Medicaid confinement of the surviving spouse, the home becomes subject to recovery. In some states, if the surviving spouse is still living in the home after the death of the recipient, Medicaid will forgive the debt and not come after the property with a lien. Also, in all states, a home below a certain market value will be exempt from recovery.

Medicaid (Medi-Cal) Gifting Rules

Provisions of the 2006 Deficit Reduction Act have made it extremely difficult to give away assets in order to accelerate qualification for Medicaid benefits. New look back rules require any gift or so-called "transfer for less than value," within 60 months of a Medicaid community waiver or nursing home stay to be counted as a resource for Medicaid qualification. This rule also applies to irrevocable trusts. Revocable trusts are not considered an asset transfer. Any applications for Medicaid benefits within this five year window will require a penalty that withholds benefits for a certain number of months based on the amount of the gift.

Here's how it works. Suppose Mary gives her daughter her $120,000 residence one year before entering a nursing home. It takes Mary 5 months in a nursing home before she has spent her remaining liquid resources down to less than $2,000 at which point she would normally become eligible for Medicaid. But she still must incur a penalty period or sanction because the $120,000 transfer occurred within 5 years.

The penalty period is determined by dividing the gifted resources by the average Medicaid reimbursement rate in the state, which in this example is $3,000 per month. The result, in this case, is a period of 40 months in which someone other than Medicaid pays for care. In this case it may be Mary's daughter. Her daughter can also transfer the title to the house back to Mary and avoid a penalty.

The penalty period starts on the date of Medicaid approval. Someone must pay for Mary's long term care costs for almost 4 years before Medicaid will take over. The gifting penalty does not mean that some planning for transferring assets can occur to preserve those assets from Medicaid.

It is best to work with a Medicaid professional or elder law attorney when contemplating gifts, going through a spend down or setting up trusts to avoid Medicaid look back and recovery. Even under the new rules some gifting is possible.

Medicaid (Medi-Cal) Home Care and Community Services
In 1981 the Medicaid Home and Community-Based Services (HCBS) Waiver program was passed by Congress. This allowed for Medicaid to pay for home health aids and personal care services in the home. States are also allowed to establish programs for care in facilities or settings other than nursing homes. In order to provide these programs, the states have to apply for and receive dollar grants for "waivers" to the Medicaid requirement for nursing home care.

The Centers for Medicare and Medicaid Services (CMS) are also experimenting with direct grant programs to states that bypass the waiver programs. Recently, Congress has authorized money for direct payment programs for home care and assisted living that also bypasses the waiver requirements. The Deficit Reduction Act of 2006 also gave states greater latitude in providing alternative services other than nursing homes.

Your local area agency on aging can give you a complete list of alternative or waiver services offered by your state and how to apply for them.

Federal Medicaid qualification for these alternative programs is the same as for the nursing home, but the individual state may apply even stricter rules for qualifying. Medicaid also recognizes that a person staying in the home to receive care and not going into a nursing home, must still pay utilities, cost of upkeep and so forth and so gives a monthly housing allowance of up to $495 a month.

Final Note
As a general rule, government programs will not pay for long term care unless there is a medical need. The exception is Medicaid, and that requires impoverishment and in most states means confinement in a nursing home.

A few other government programs will pay for home care that is nonmedical under certain conditions. The care recipient must be low income and have virtually no assets.

Medicaid rules and qualifications are so complex that it is advised to work with an elder law attorney or other expert before applying. Once you have qualified for Medicaid, you are eligible for a broad range of services. Unlike Medicare, there are no premiums or deductibles or time of use stipulations. Fees by doctors, nursing homes, and other providers are set, and you are not charged more for the difference.

Veterans Long Term Care Benefits
The Department of Veterans Affairs provides three types of long term care services for veterans.

1. VA Healthcare System Long Term Care Services
These services are for individuals who have substantial service-connected disabilities, who are receiving VA Pension or who are considered low income. Services include possible free medical care, possible free prescription drugs, orthotics and prosthetics, home renovation grants for disabilities, home care, assisted living, domiciliary care, nursing home care, and a possible host of other long term care benefits.

These services are not available to all veterans in the health care system. Availability depends on the local medical center's funds, the nature of the disability or whether the veteran is considered very low income.

2. State Veterans Homes
The majority of these homes offer nursing care but some may offer assisted living or domiciliary care. The Department of Veterans Affairs in conjunction with the states, helps build and support state veterans homes. Money is provided to help with construction and a federal subsidy of $71.42 (2008) a day is provided for each veteran using state veterans nursing home services. These homes are generally available for most veterans and sometimes their spouses and in some cases so-called "Goldstar parents." Veterans homes are run by the states, sometimes with the help of contract management. There may be waiting lists in some states.

3. Disability Income for Veterans Who Served on Active Duty
The first of these disability incomes is called Compensation and is designed to award the veteran a certain amount of money to compensate for potential loss of income in the private sector due to a disability or injury or illness incurred in the service. In order to receive Compensation, a veteran has to have evidence of a service-connected disability. Most veterans who are receiving this benefit were awarded an amount based on a percentage of disability when they left the service.

However, some veterans may have record of being exposed to extreme cold, having an inservice, nondisabling injury, having tropical diseases or tuberculosis or other incidents or exposures that at the time may not have caused any disability but years later have resulted in medical problems. These people can apply to see if they could receive a benefit. In addition, some veterans may be receiving Compensation but their condition has worsened, and they can reapply for a larger amount based on a higher disability rating. There is generally no income or asset test for most forms of Compensation, and the benefit is nontaxable.

The second disability income benefit is called Pension. Pension is also called "Veterans Aid and Attendance Benefit." It is available to all active-duty veterans who served at least 90 days during a period of war. Applicants younger than age 65 must be totally disabled or a patient in a nursing home. Veterans younger than 65, receiving Social Security disability, have a lesser burden of proof. Proof of disability is not required for applicants age 65 or over. Age is evidence by itself of disability.

The purpose of this benefit is to provide supplemental income to disabled or older veterans who have a low income. If the veteran's income exceeds the Pension amount, then there is no award. However, income can be adjusted for unreimbursed medical expenses, and this allows veterans with household incomes larger than the Pension amount to qualify for a monthly benefit. For example, a veteran household earning $6,000 a month could still qualify for Pension under the right circumstances.

There is also an asset test to qualify for Pension. The primary residence, most personal property and automobiles are exempt from this asset test.

Compensation and Pension claims are submitted on the same form and VA will consider paying either benefit. Generally, for applications associated with the cost of home care, assisted living or nursing home care, the Pension benefit is more money.

There are also several death benefit variations of the two disability incomes for single surviving spouses or dependent minor children or adult dependent children.

Death Pension is one of these benefits and is a lesser amount based on the same rules for applying for a living Pension claimant. In other words, the deceased veteran must have met the rules for Pension -- with the exception of being totally disabled or over age 65 -- or have been receiving Pension in order for his or her spouse to receive the lesser benefit. In addition, in order to keep receiving the benefit, the surviving spouse must remain single.

Asset tests and income tests also apply to a death Pension, and, basically, all the rules are the same for obtaining the benefit as with the living veteran.

Benefit levels are lower for a surviving spouse when compared to a single veteran. For example, a single veteran with no dependent children is entitled to an MAPR (Maximum Allowable Pension Rate) of $11,181 without aid and attendance and $18,654 with aid and attendance. In comparison, a surviving spouse is entitled to an MAPR of $7,498 without aid and attendance and $11,985 with aid and attendance.

There are applications and forms required to submit for approval to receive VA benefits. Medical and income qualifications apply. The most comprehensive site on the Internet, everything you wanted to know about this benefit is found at www.veteransaidbenefit.org

Planning Strategies -- Preserving Assets and Creating Cash for Care Costs

VA Benefit Alternative to Spending Savings or Selling a House
Estimates are that as much as 33% of the population over age 65 could qualify for the VA pension benefit when the need for long term care arises. This benefit can pay up to $1,843 of the cost of long term care in addition to existing income.

Veterans age 65 and over, who served during a period of war, and their surviving spouses, are eligible recipients..

VA considers this a benefit for low income recipients. A special provision in calculating the benefit can allow households earning as much as $3,000-$4,000 a month to receive the income.

Unfortunately, the claims form and instructions do not disclose how to obtain the maximum benefit. This usually requires a specialist who is familiar with the claims procedure in order to avoid a denial or reduced award for higher income applicants. Most communities have a specialist who is familiar with this benefit and the application process.

Having an additional $1,843 a month can make the difference between selling the house to move to a facility or receiving paid care from a home care agency and remaining in the home. Also, the money can be used to protect savings from the cost of assisted living. Finally, the benefit can be used to defray the cost of Medicaid spend down. Go to www.veteransaidbenefit.org for more information.

Converting Assets to Income to Qualify for Veterans Benefit
Some veterans or their spouses or surviving spouses are prevented from receiving the pension benefit because their assets exceed $80,000. Assets can be gifted outright or converted to income through an annuity, but care must be taken to structure this properly in case there might be a subsequent application for Medicaid. Obtaining advice from a specialist who understands Medicaid and the veterans benefit is extremely important. Go to www.veteransaidbenefit.org for more information.

VA Pension or Medicaid to Pay Family Members for Care

Both Medicaid and the "Veterans Aid and Attendance Benefit" allow a long term care recipient to pay members of the family to provide legitimate care. This can be an effective way of recognizing the sacrifice of family members who care for their loved ones by transferring assets to them in the form of payments for care.

Otherwise -- primarily with Medicaid -- money cannot be directly gifted to family members without creating an eligibility penalty. In addition, with the Veterans Aid and Attendance Program, money paid to family members can usually be replaced in the form of additional income to the veteran household. Go to www.veteransaidbenefit.org for more information.

Asset Transfers to Qualify for VA Aid and Attendance Benefit

Even though 1/3 of seniors could qualify for the aid and attendance benefit, they must meet an income and asset test. It is not usually difficult to meet the income test because of the allowed deduction from income for the high cost of long term care.

These ongoing care costs can be subtracted from income to meet that test. However, assets in excess of $80,000 will disqualify applicants. And any level of assets below $80,000 could block a claim depending on the decision of the VA employee processing that claim. A home, vehicle and personal property are exempt from this asset test.

Applicants can give away assets or convert those assets to income and VA will not penalize them as with Medicaid. And unlike Medicaid there is no look back penalty period either. But these transfers have to be done correctly. It is also extremely important that any transfers meet Medicaid transfer rules, since it is highly possible that the VA beneficiary might also need to apply for Medicaid inside the five-year look back for asset transfers.

A consultant who understands these benefits should be contacted to make sure transfers are done properly. Go to www.veteransaidbenefit.org for more information.

Dovetailing Veterans Benefits with Medicaid

VA rules require halting the payment of pension benefits if a single veteran or surviving spouse is eligible for Medicaid and living in a nursing home. The single beneficiary can receive only $90 a month in Pension benefit.

However, if there is a spouse at home or if the veteran or the spouse are going through a spend down process to qualify for Medicaid, then the pension benefit can be helpful in preserving assets or providing more income for the spouse at home. But dovetailing the planning for getting a pension award can be complicated by the gifting rules for Medicaid. It is extremely important to work with someone who understands both benefits such that qualifying for the VA pension does not disqualify one for Medicaid.

Medicaid Spend down for Funeral Trust

Medicaid will allow a Medicaid applicant to transfer a certain amount of assets into a trust that will pay for funeral and/or burial costs at death. In many states the maximum allowable amount is $15,000. These trusts are often funded with special life insurance policies. The trust must be irrevocable and meet Medicaid rules for such trusts.

More about Medicaid Annuities

If one spouse in a couple needs long term care costs to be covered by Medicaid, the couple must divide combined assets in half and the spouse needing care must spend his or her half of the assets down to less than $2,000 remaining. This loss of assets may reduce the standard of living for the healthy spouse at home.

Medicaid will allow the spouse needing care to convert his or her share of the assets into an income annuity that belongs to the healthy spouse. This legal strategy provides the healthy spouse with more income and avoids the impoverishment imposed by the spend down. These annuities must meet strict rules imposed by Medicaid and an expert in this area should be sought out.

In the past, advisers also recommended these income annuities for single Medicaid beneficiaries in order to transfer some of the spend down assets to members of the family at the death of the annuitant. The Deficit Reduction Act of 2006 changed the rules for these single

Medicaid beneficiary annuities and did away with their use as a planning tool for asset transfers. Under certain circumstances partial transfers can still be done using a Medicaid beneficiary income annuity called a "half-a-loaf" transfer. As with a spouse annuity, an expert should be sought in order to make sure this is done properly.

Medicaid Anticipation Deferred Annuity
Money can be invested in deferred annuities anticipating the eventual annuitization (conversion into guaranteed income) for Medicaid purposes. Many practitioners set up these investments inside of living trusts which also avoid probate. These deferred annuities should be designed so that the money can be turned into a guaranteed income stream for either spouse of a couple. The income stream must go to the healthy spouse -- the one not requiring Medicaid assistance.

Medicaid or VA Benefits and an Unoccupied Home
In most states Medicaid will allow a single Medicaid beneficiary to leave his or her primary residence unoccupied while that person is residing in a facility. Not living in the home does not disqualify a person from receiving Medicaid in most states. VA takes the same attitude when someone is receiving the aid and attendance benefit in a facility.

Any rental income from an unoccupied home must be counted as income for both programs and could create a problem with eligibility. The family could also be tempted to sell the residence which would then create assets that would disqualify the recipient for both programs -- Medicaid and VA. Finally, family members might transfer the title to the property which would also disqualify the Medicaid recipient and cause problems with the VA benefit.

A specialist in this area of expertise should be consulted to learn the best strategy to deal with an unoccupied home.

When the Value of the House Exceeds $500,000 ($750,000 in Some States)
Any single person applying for Medicaid in a facility, and owning a house worth more than $500,000 ($750,000 in some states) is ineligible for Medicaid assistance. This is only the case where the house is not occupied by a spouse or other qualifying dependent.

Apparently, the intent of this rule is to have the house sold and the proceeds used towards paying the facility care before Medicaid needs to take over. This is a new rule and its application in practice is going to be difficult for some applicants to handle due to a number of underlying problems associated with disposing of the property.

You should contact a specialist who can help with the problems associated with disposing of the property, reducing its value or otherwise finding a way around this rule.

Transferring Title to Avoid Medicaid Recovery
As far as we know, Medicaid is the only government entitlement program that attempts to go after a beneficiary's home after that person dies. Medicare, Social Security, disaster relief, crop subsidies, income assistance and a host of other government support programs do not place liens against someone's property after they die to repay the government for the money it spent on that person's behalf.

A great amount of the money for government support programs does not come from beneficiary contributions but directly from the general budget. This includes Medicare and Social Security. Yet, Medicaid appears to be the only program that tries to recover these general budget dollars.

As unfair and inequitable as Medicaid recovery is, it is still a reality that must be dealt with. There are legal ways to keep property out of the hands of Medicaid recovery.

When one spouse ends up in a nursing home under Medicaid and the other spouse remains at home, the Medicaid spouse should transfer his or her interest on the title to the spouse at home. The title can then be transferred through a trust or directly to the family to avoid Medicaid recovery should the healthy spouse eventually need care as long as it is beyond the 5 year look back period.

Here's another strategy. A very common situation is for one of the children to live in the home of the parent and take care of that parent. If that situation has occurred for two years or longer, and it can be shown that the care provided by a child living in the house of the parent has kept a parent from applying for Medicaid, there is a special rule that allows the family to keep the house away from Medicaid recovery.

Having met the conditions above, the parent needing Medicaid can transfer the title to the caregiving child. This is an exempt transaction and will not disqualify the parent from receiving Medicaid.

For both of these situations, an elder law attorney should be consulted to make sure it is done right and to help provide the proper paperwork for approval.

Don't Sell the House but Find Other Strategies for Nursing Home Costs

Some states allow a single Medicaid recipient in a nursing home to retain possession of a personal residence even though the recipient is not living in it. Family members are often too eager to sell the property to help pay for the nursing home. In those states that allow it, the home need not be sold. Possession of a vacant home will not prevent the parent from receiving Medicaid.

This allows the parent to receive Medicaid without spending down the entire value derived from the sale of the home. It also allows the possibility of renting the home and applying the rent -- which is a Medicaid requirement -- towards the cost of care. Both of these strategies can help retain the value of the home. This is because the amount that Medicaid pays for the nursing home, possibly reduced by rental income, may never equal the equity value of the home.

After the death of the parent, Medicaid recovery against the property may only demand a fraction of the value of the home. On the other hand, selling the home and going through a spend down process could result in losing the entire value of the home.

An elder law attorney should be consulted to make sure this is a viable option in your state.

Investment Strategies

There are a number of strategies to maximize the value of retirement savings accounts and thereby help cover the cost of long term care.

Even for older people, there should be some portion of the retirement savings invested in stocks. A common recommendation is about 50% stock mutual funds and about 50% in CDs or conservative bond funds. Since many people are living 25 to 35 years beyond retirement, prudent investment strategies can make a big difference in the outcome of that retirement.

Research into strategies for taking money out of retirement savings accounts also shows that the proper withdrawal strategies can make a big difference in preserving remaining assets.

Investment advisers or retirement planning counselors are well worth the money for consultation.

Deferred Annuities Provide Tax Advantages and Potentially Better Earnings

The appeal of deferred annuities is the deferral of taxes on earnings until money is withdrawn or the annuity is converted into a guaranteed income stream. Deferred annuities can also avoid probate if the owner chooses not to create a living trust for this purpose. As a general rule, annuities have the potential of producing an average yearly rate of return somewhat better than a bank CD or savings account. Annuity returns also tend to be more stable than short-term savings.

Life Insurance for Long Term Care Planning

Life insurance companies have become more competitive in recent years for policies issued on people over age 70. Good health is still a major consideration for low premiums but policies have been redesigned to provide more death benefit and less cash value. Some term policies and certain universal life permanent policies are designed to provide a guaranteed death benefit up to age 95 with a guaranteed premium and no cash value at all. This design generally results in more death benefit for each premium dollar. Also, policies designed for couples -- second-to-die policies -- can provide a significant amount of insurance for a one-time single premium even if one of the partners is in very poor health.

An important concept to consider is that single premium life policies, with no cash value and purchased for estate planning purposes, many years in advance of applying for Medicaid, can be a valuable planning tool if the need for Medicaid arises. Medicaid does not apply the death benefit of a life insurance policy to the asset spend down rule. But the cash value of any policy that has more than $1,500 in cash will count towards the asset test and could disqualify a Medicaid applicant.

As an example, a person could have $1 million of life insurance with cash value less than $1,500 and it would not prevent that person from receiving Medicaid. However, cash value of more than $1,500 in this example will apply toward the asset test.

It is important to know, for planning purposes, that people who apply for Medicaid and <u>then transfer assets to a life insurance policy, while they are going through spend down</u>, could be in violation of their state's Medicaid transfer rules and such an act may disqualify the applicant. Life insurance as a Medicaid planning tool must be done many years in advance of applying for Medicaid.

Life insurance can be used as an alternative for funding the cost of long term care. If someone planning for the eventuality of long term care is concerned about losing assets that would normally be passed on to the children or be needed by a surviving spouse, that person can invest a portion of those assets in life insurance and leverage a death benefit payout -- sometimes for up to $3.00 in death benefit for every $1.00 in single premium. The death benefit is also income tax-free.

A person creating such an estate can then use remaining assets for long term care needs in the future but still be assured that the children or a surviving spouse will receive an inheritance at death through the life insurance. And, as discussed above, if the money runs out and Medicaid has to start picking up the costs, a single premium life insurance policy with less than $1,500 cash value will not disqualify the applicant owning the policy

Another use for life insurance for the elderly is in paying the cost of final expenses such as funeral and burial. A number of companies will issue policies without any health questions for people who may not have very long to live. Most of these policies will provide little or no death benefit in the first two years after issue and so there is some risk, but most companies will also return the premiums paid if death occurs in the first two years.

IRA or 401(k) Income Life Annuity to Buy Life Insurance
Tax qualified investments such as IRAs, 401(k)s, Tax Sheltered Annuities and other tax favored plans are great for saving taxes while one is working but many seniors find they don't need that money during retirement and they may want to pass on some of this tax sheltered money to their children.

New "stretch IRA" rules have made it easier to reduce the immediate tax burden on these transfers at death but income tax that was deferred must still be paid. The income tax on these transferred assets can eat up a significant portion of the investment because it is calculated at ordinary income tax rates.

One way to create a tax-free transfer at death is to convert the IRA, TSA or 401(k) into a life annuity income while the owner is alive. Part of the income is used to purchase a life insurance policy that would equal the amount of money in the IRA -- intended as an inheritance. A life insurance death benefit is income tax-free and thus the loss of a significant part of the account to taxes has been avoided.

Tax Strategies
If you are investing in mutual funds, then tax free bonds and index funds are going to produce the least taxable income. In the case of municipal tax free bond funds, dividends are not taxable for state income taxes and possibly federal taxes, and only capital gains from the sale or appreciation of the underlying bonds are taxable.

Investment in the right kind of tax free bond funds may result in savings on both state and federal income taxes. Index funds typically produce less taxable income due to a low turnover in the stock holdings and resulting low capital gains earnings.

Individuals who own property that has high deferred capital gains, have a number of tax strategies available. One is a tax-free exchange to a new similar property. Another very common strategy for older investors is to give the property to a charitable organization using a charitable remainder trust and avoid most taxes altogether. There are a number of strategies that can be used based on charitable gifting.

The most popular vehicle for reducing estate taxes is a trust designed for that purpose. There are also gifting strategies along the way to reduce the size of the estate.

There are myriad trust arrangements to transfer assets to the next generation and reduce such taxes as generation skipping taxes and other potential taxes. Some planners use partnerships as a means to transfer assets. Other planners might use arrangements with life interests.

You should always stay in touch with a qualified estate planning attorney and/or CPA who specializes in these areas.

Restructure Insurance and Eliminate Costs
One way for healthy seniors to save costs is to switch from traditional Medicare with a supplement to a Medicare Advantage plan. In some cases seniors can save $2,000 to $3,000 a year. These savings should be retained in a bank account since Medicare advantage plans require more upfront deductibles or co-pays for hospital care or long term care than traditional Medicare with a supplement.

Many seniors have cash value life insurance policies that might be paying for themselves without future premiums. This possibility should be investigated.

Some people on Medicare are buying health supplement policies to pay for cancer or intensive care. Since most people on Medicare are adequately covered for cancer or intensive care, these policies may not be necessary and premiums could be saved.

Many seniors do not take the time to reevaluate homeowners or auto insurance to see if money can be saved. For instance the auto policy may be covering a vehicle that has long since lost its value but yet the policy may have low deductibles for comprehensive and collusion.

In the event of an accident, the insurance company may only pay for the replacement value of the vehicle. The low deductibles may offer no benefit for repair or new replacement. Money could be saved by restructuring the policy.

Other insurance policies should be reevaluated as to their usefulness and a decision made whether to keep them or save the premiums.

Use of Trusts for Other than Estate Tax Planning

A common trust called a living trust, is often used to transfer property, avoiding probate. As a general rule, these trusts are useful in states that have high probate costs. In states where probate has been simplified and the cost reduced, these trusts may not be as useful. But they do allow transfer without public disclosure as opposed to the probate process. It may also be possible in those states with deficient Medicaid recovery rules that this type of trust could escape Medicaid recovery against the personal residence.

Living trusts are also useful where family members may not be reliable administrators of the estate. For various reasons, the trust maker may prefer to have a third party administer the transfer of estate assets, and in addition carry out wishes that would only be appropriate for a noninvolved trust administrator. In many cases allowing a family member to handle investments or the disbursement of trust assets could be a disaster. Due to inexperience or incompetence, assets could be dissipated.

Banks have trust departments for this purpose, but we recommend a professional trust administrative company that specializes in this area. A trust company is typically more adept and cheaper at administering trust instructions and managing assets. In fact, some individuals actually use the investment arms of trust management companies instead of using brokers or other investment advisers to manage their investments. The trust company often does a better job. In other words the trust company can often manage funds as a separate function not involving the administration of a trust.

In some situations, trusts can be used to gift assets to family members and preserve those assets from Medicaid spend down. In addition, trusts can be used to reduce assets to below $80,000 to qualify for the VA pension. In these cases an elder law attorney or estate planning attorney can be invaluable in helping the family preserve assets or create more income.

Reverse Mortgage Life Insurance Strategy
Some older people don't like the idea of doing a reverse mortgage because they feel they are robbing their heirs of an inheritance or there is something inherently wrong in using up the equity in the home.

A useful strategy that typically appeals to these people is to take part of the reverse mortgage proceeds and buy a life insurance policy that has a death benefit equal to the amount of equity taken out by the reverse mortgage. A couple in their 70s could possibly buy an insurance policy for $50,000 that would pay $150,000 at the last death.

The reverse mortgage produces $150,000 in available funds. After buying the insurance, there is $100,000 in funds still available. But when the couple dies the family inherits $150,000 tax-free to replace the loss in equity to the reverse mortgage.

Reverse Mortgage Long Term Care Insurance Strategy
Using the same reverse mortgage example above, the couple could leave the money from the reverse mortgage in a line of credit and draw out enough every year to pay a $5,000 annual premium for a long term care insurance policy for both of them. When the time comes for long term care, the policy allows them to save their assets, including the money in the line of credit which is growing with interest.

STEP 3

Using Long Term Care Professionals

*Using professional help relieves stress,
reduces conflict, and saves time and money*

Long Term Care Planning Requires a Team Approach

Long term care services are complicated and provider contacts are fragmented throughout the community. For the majority of Americans, eldercare becomes a frustrating do-it-yourself process. This approach is unnecessary. Using care professionals is the most cost effective and efficient way to provide help for a loved one.

Hiring professional advisers or providers to help with long term care is no different than using professionals to help with other complex issues such as car repairs, dealing with taxes, dealing with legal problems, or needing trained employees to help run a business.

With their education and training, long term care professionals also bring experience that only comes from dealing with countless hands-on, caregiving challenges. You should use this valuable experience.

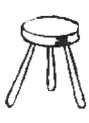 In much the same way that a three legged stool needs all three legs to be useful, the care planning approach needs at least three key entities in order to be successful. It needs **YOU, LONG TERM CARE PROFESSIONALS**, and **GOVERNMENT LONG TERM CARE PROGRAMS**. Learn more in this chapter about how these three elements work together in planning for long term care.

An Example of How Team Care Planning Can Work

Mary is taking care of her aging husband at home. He has diabetes and is overweight. Because of the diabetes, her husband has severe neuropathy in his legs and feet and it is difficult for him to walk. He also has diabetic retinopathy and, therefore, cannot see very well. She has to be careful that he does not injure his feet, since the last time that happened he was in the hospital for four weeks with a severe infection. She is having difficulty helping him out of bed and with dressing and using the bathroom. She relies heavily on her son, who lives nearby, to help her manage her husband's care.

On the advice of a friend, Mary is told about a professional care manager, Sharon Brown. The cost of an initial assessment and care plan from the care manager is $300.00. Mary thinks she has the situation under control and $300.00 for someone from the outside to come in and tell her how to deal with her situation seems ridiculous.

One day Mary is trying to lift her husband and injures her back severely. She is bedridden and cannot care for her husband. Her son, who works fulltime, now has two parents to care for. On the advice of the same friend, he decides to bring in Sharon Brown and pay her fee himself.

Sharon does a thorough assessment of the family's needs. She arranges for Mary's doctor to order Medicare home care during Mary's recovery. Therapists come in and help Mary with exercises and advice on lifting. Sharon advertises for and finds a private individual who is willing to live in the home for a period of time to help Mary with her recovery and watch over her husband. Sharon makes sure the new caregiver is reliable and honest and that taxes are paid for the employment. Sharon enlists the support of the local area agency on aging and makes sure all services available are provided for the family.

Sharon also calls a meeting with Mary's family and explains to them the care needs and how they need to commit to help with those needs. Sharon makes arrangements to rent or purchase medical equipment for lifting, moving and easier use of the bathroom facilities. Medicare will pay much of this cost.

Sharon suggests using a geriatric care physician she works closely with to help Mary in the care of her husband. The geriatrician meets with Mary and her husband and spends a great deal of time explaining the proper treatment and care of elderly with diabetes. He rearranges medications and puts Mary's husband on a new insulin regimen to better control his blood sugar. The physician starts a strict diet and insists on weight loss and exercise. The previous doctor seemed more interested in treating symptoms than in changing lifestyles. The geriatric physician feels that Mary's husband has a chance of improving his health with proper treatment.

Sharon also works closely with an elder law attorney and a financial planner who specializes in the elderly. The attorney prepares documents for the family including powers of attorney, a living will and advice on preserving Mary's remaining assets. The financial planner recommends a reverse mortgage specialist to help Mary and her husband tap unused assets in their home's equity.

Some reverse mortgage proceeds are used to pay off debt. The remaining proceeds are converted into income with a single premium immediate annuity in order to provide Mary adequate income when her husband is gone and she loses one of the Social Security payments.

With the help of the care manager, Mary's life and future have been significantly improved. Her husband as well, if he adheres to the care plan, may end up having a better quality of life for his remaining years.

In the above example, medical services, legal and financial services, government aging services, and government Medicare came together to provide improved long term care services with several bonus helps for Mary and her husband that she was not aware of.

We provide in this chapter a list of long term care professionals with a summary of their services. You can locate each of these professionals in your area on www.longtermcarelink.net.

The following professional service providers or advisers are discussed in detail in the ensuing pages of this section of the book.

1. Professional Care Manager

Also known as Geriatric Care Managers, Elder Care or Aging Care Managers, a Professional Care Manager represents a growing trend to help full time, employed family caregivers provide care for loved ones. Care managers are expert in assisting caregivers, friends or family members find government-paid and private resources to help with long term care decisions.

They are professionals, trained to evaluate and recommend care for the aged. They can be a nurse, social worker, psychologist, or gerontologist who specializes in assessing the abilities and needs of the elderly. Below is a partial list of what a care manager or geriatric care manager might do:

- Assess the level and type of care needed and develop a care plan.
- Take steps to start the care plan and keep it functioning.
- Make sure care is in a safe and disability friendly environment.
- Resolve family conflicts and other issues with long term care.
- Become an advocate for the care recipient and the caregiver.
- Manage care for a loved one for out-of-town families.
- Conduct ongoing assessments to implement changes in care.
- Oversee and direct care provided at home.
- Coordinate the efforts of key support systems.
- Provide personal counseling.
- Help with Medicaid qualification and application.
- Arrange for services of legal and financial advisors.
- Provide placement in assisted living facilities or nursing homes.
- Monitor the care received in a nursing home or in assisted living.
- Assist with the monitoring of medications.
- Find appropriate solutions to avoid a crisis.
- Coordinate medical appointments and medical information.
- Provide transportation to medical appointments
- Assist families in positive decision making
- Develop care plans for older loved ones not now needing care

For those who desire to remain in the home, the care manager can help make that a reality and keep the care recipient away from a premature admittance into a care facility.

But the care manager can also help in the other direction. Oftentimes, the family is attempting to keep a loved one at home when that is not the best situation. For many and various reasons, care in the home may be impossible.

For example, consider the family where all family members are employed full time and both mom and dad need intensive care at home. There is also not enough money to pay for caregivers to come into the home. In an attempt to cover the situation, the family trades off taking care of mom and dad in the morning and in the evening and on weekends. But they simply can't attend properly to the needs.

A care manager will have a better and more objective perspective of the situation. In this case an assisted living facility would be a much better choice. If there is not enough money, then a Medicaid facility may be the only choice.

Also take the example of an individual who has Alzheimer's and has become difficult to manage. It just may not be possible for a caregiver in the home to deal with it, but because of stubbornness or lack of proper judgment, the caregiver is trying to cope. Again, a care manager knows what to do and can help in this situation by recommending a different care environment.

When trying to arrange care for a parent who lives in another state, securing the services of a care manger can be your greatest asset. A manger, who is in your parent's area, will assess your loved one's needs and communicate to you the best care options. The care manager will also be your eyes, ears and legs in helping you take care of your loved one by long-distance.

Care managers can charge anywhere from $50.00 an hour to $200.00 an hour, or they may charge a flat fee for a care assessment and plan and then hourly for services beyond that. Cost is usually covered from personal funds. Long term care insurance may cover the cost of an assessment, as many policies will pay $250.00 to $300.00 for a care assessment. Policy language usually refers to this as care coordination. Medicaid or Medicare will not pay for this service, but an area agency on aging may offer case management for certain low income or socially disadvantaged individuals.

Find out the care manager's billing policy. Some will bill weekly or monthly and others bill at the end of their assessment or service. There may also be charges that are not in their hourly fee. These may be mileage, phone charges, etc. If another type of professional, like a doctor or lawyer, is brought in by the care manager, these other specialists will also charge for their services. Make sure you are notified before they are brought in and their fees are approved.

When you are comfortable with the arrangement, get everything in writing. This will insure what you and the care manager expect from each other.

How do you locate a care manager?

- Local yellow page listings may be under Home Care, Home Health Services, Senior Services
- State aging services or Senior Centers may have information on finding care managers in your area
- Your physician or local hospital social worker

The National Association of Professional Geriatric Care Managers has a referral network throughout the country. **(520) 881-8008** You can locate a care manager in your area on www.longtermcarelink.net

2. Geriatric Medical Services

Geriatricians or other Practitioners in Aging Medicine
Geriatricians are doctors or nurse practitioners who specialize in treating older people. In seeking medical professional help, the elderly or their family should attempt to discover geriatric care specialists in their area. If that is not possible an effort should be made to locate a geriatric clinic in the area.

Geriatric clinics are becoming more popular, and even though the doctors who staff them may not always be geriatric physicians, they are likely to be well aware of the problems associated with treating elderly people. Many geriatric clinics include a team of specialists to help older people. Here are some of the specialists who may be available in a geriatric clinic:

- Geriatrician
- Nurse
- Social worker
- Nutritionist
- Physical therapist
- Occupational therapist
- Consultant pharmacist
- Geropsychiatrist

If there are no geriatricians or geriatric clinics in the area, an attempt should be made to find those doctors who specialize in elderly care. This can be done by making phone calls to various doctors' offices or by checking in the Yellow Pages. It is to the older person's benefit to find a doctor who understands aging and how to treat older people. Proper geriatric health care might even help relieve the amount of care needed for an older person by improving health and reducing disabilities.

House Call Doctors
Many doctors are returning to the practice of medicine a hundred years ago and are making house calls. Health insurance plans, including Medicare, will now reimburse a doctor and possibly a staff member, if test equipment is involved, to visit homebound patients in their homes.

To qualify for a home visit, the patient must have to experience great difficulty in leaving the home in order meet with the doctor in his or her office. This does not, however, mean the care recipient need be totally disabled. It simply means that transportation requirements or help needed to get to a doctor might be very expensive or difficult to provide or the patient's safety might be jeopardized by leaving the home.

Doctors are willing to visit in the home and provide service because they are paid more money by health insurance providers to compensate them for their time and their loss of efficiency in meeting patients in their offices. Probably the insurance providers reason that the additional cost of meeting with patients at home, before major medical problems evolve, is more cost effective than paying for ambulances and treatment in emergency rooms.

Physicians Orders For Life Sustaining Treatment (POLST)
A POLST form is a physician's order that records your wishes for resuscitation, use of antibiotics, artificially administered fluids, and nutrition.

How it works:
Your physician or nurse practitioner records your preferences and signs the POLST form. This becomes your prescription for treatment and is binding legally for your wishes, even if you are mentally unable to communicate when that time comes.

You can change the order at any time. A copy should be kept with your physician as well as a family member and yourself. In the case of a 911 call for an emergency, the form must go with you so they know your wishes. Otherwise, the emergency attendants are required to apply all lifesaving procedures.

You can state the amount of care you want on this form. For example, if you do not want a feeding tube, you can state that, or you may want minimum and temporary use of a feeding tube. Official POLST forms can be found on the internet under your state's department of health website or may be procured from your physician.

3. Professional Home Care Services

For the elderly, who need long term care services, the choice to stay in their home almost always requires some type of help and service from others. There are many options to choose from in home care and the choice is usually made by the degree of personal or medical need.

It is important to educate yourself on the types of home care services before choosing one. There are many different services becoming available, from licensed home care companies, house cleaning services and errand services to companion services.

State Licensed Home Health Agency
A home health agency that is a state licensed company and is Medicare certified is used for homebound patients requiring medical attention or physical therapy. You may be referred to this type of agency upon discharge from a nursing home rehabilitation stay or more likely by your doctor when the need arises for medical aid as well as personal aid in your home.

These companies must meet legal and operating standards set by the state department of health. Your local area on aging or health department can provide you with the names of home health agencies that are licensed and Medicare certified.

Home health agencies provide all medical personnel and services necessary for support in the home. Some of these are:

- Registered Nurse or Licensed Practical Nurse
- Physical, speech and occupational therapists
- Social workers
- Individual and family counseling
- Medication training and compliance
- Management of IVs, wound dressing
- Blood pressure monitoring
- Diet and meal planning
- Bathing, dressing, light housekeeping

The chart below shows the type of help or skilled need most required from a home health agency.

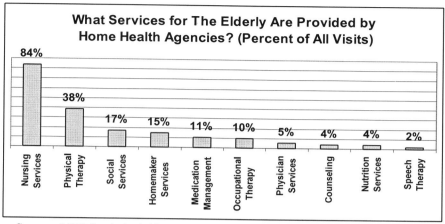

Source: 2005 Statistical Abstract of The United States, Health And Nutrition

Most agencies hire, train, and supervise their personnel. They work with your doctor (or their doctor) in seeing you get the right medical treatment and supervision. They may also, as needed, secure the services of professionals such as infusion therapists or medical equipment companies. They can be your most valuable aid in staying in your home.

As an example, when Jill's mother broke her hip, she spent a week in the hospital recovering. When she was released, she still could not walk or take care of herself. As she was going home to live with Jill and not go to a nursing home for rehabilitation, her doctor prescribed a state licensed, Medicare home health service.

The home health care company worked with Jill to make her mother's room and living conditions comfortable. They secured an air bed that relieved the pressure from bed sores her mother had developed in the hospital. Nurses were assigned twice a day to come and treat her wounds. Aids came twice a day to bath, dress, and prepare her mom for the day and for night comfort. Even though her room was in Jill's home, they cleaned it and changed her bed daily. They worked with Jill on diet and medications. A physical therapist came in twice a week to work with her mother's mobility.

Jill's mother was soon able to sit in a chair and walk without help. The support from the home health care made it possible for Jill to have her mother stay in her home until her death and relieved the much of the burden of caregiving. Medicare paid for almost all of it.

Another bonus from the professional companies is that they take care of the paper work, taxes, Medicare forms, etc. Also, they make sure that the people show up to do their job.

Non-Medical Home Care Services
These providers represent a rapidly growing trend to allow people needing help with long term care to remain in their homes or in the community instead of going to a care facility. The services offered may include:

- companionship
- grooming and dressing
- recreational activities
- incontinent care
- handyman services
- teeth brushing
- medication reminders
- bathing or showering
- light housekeeping
- meal preparation
- respite for family caregivers
- errands and shopping
- reading email or letters
- overseeing home deliveries
- dealing with vendors
- transportation services
- changing linens
- laundry and ironing
- organizing closets
- care of house plants
- 24-hour emergency response
- family counseling
- phone call checks

A search of your local yellow pages under "Home Health Agencies" will reveal that a large number of the advertised providers are personal care or non-medical home health companies. This causes some confusion since the yellow pages choose the same classification to list non-medical and traditional home care agencies together.

Non-medical home care agencies are different from traditional home health agencies in that they do not provide medical services or skilled services and they are not paid by Medicare.

In addition, many states do not require non-medical home care providers to license with the state health department. In some states a person desiring to start a business like this need only advertise, get a business license, and start hiring employees.

On the other hand, some states require these companies to meet the same stringent rules under which traditional home health agencies operate. This might include hiring trained employees, the use of care plans, periodic inspections by the state health department, and bonding.

If you live in a state that does not require regulation of these companies, it is important for you to check the background and history of these providers before using their services.

Another benefit for the public is that many of these companies are part of a national franchise system. There are a growing number of these home care provider franchises around the country. Being a franchise, it is more likely that you can trust the services of the company and not have to worry about theft or abuse with your loved one.

Non-medical home care services are paid for out-of-pocket, and in most cases by long term care insurance. However, some long term care insurance policies will not pay home care providers who are not licensed. If you live in a state that requires licensing of these providers the insurance should pay for their services

Privately Hired Assistant
Hiring someone to live in the home to provide 24-hour companionship or hiring a nonlicensed individual to come in daily to provide services, is another way to secure home care.

It is important to note that unlike professional home care agencies, individuals from the community do not need to be licensed by the state or be Medicare approved. You will be paying for these services yourself. You will need to do the investigating of the individual to secure someone honest, moral, and capable of performing the service you want. Where a home care agency makes sure their people will show up, if the person you have hired is ill or takes a vacation, you will be without that person.

Since you are paying a wage, you will also be responsible for taxes. These people will be on your payroll as you are their employer. The IRS has special instructions and forms to help you pay the taxes for home-based employees.

Home Telehealth
Technology has developed computer and computer cameras to help the elderly in their homes stay safe and healthy. Home telehealth -- set up by medical professionals in the home -- enables providers to monitor such things as medications and blood pressure and actually see the patient. Patient questions are answered and advice is given, while the monitoring nurse views through the video phone how his or her patient looks physically.

Home telehealth is used primarily in rural areas where long distances make visits by home care providers difficult on a regular basis. On the other hand, telehealth compensates for fewer visits by allowing these providers close monitoring and contact on a daily basis.

Payment by Medicare and Medicaid for this service is determined by each state and the rules of eligibility under homecare waivers.

To locate home care service providers who may provide telehealth in your area go to www.longtermcarelink.net.

4. Home Maintenance, Transportation & Chore Services

Many seniors who want to remain in their homes find it difficult because of a lack of transportation or because of the necessity of maintaining the home and the yard and being unable to do so.

There are numerous community and private services that provide such things as home repair, deep cleaning, remodeling, maintaining the yard, shoveling snow, transportation, and so on. Sometimes Medicaid or the local community area agency on aging will provide these services for financially needy individuals for free. For people with means there may be a charge.

There is currently a growing trend for private companies to provide these services for a fee. These companies do back ground checks, training, and supervision of their people. The company has qualified workers in all areas of home maintenance, repair, yard work, etc. Using such a company eliminates your need to do background checks, supervise, or take care of payroll. You can locate these services in your local area phone book or online at www.longtermcarelink.net

5. Home Disability Support & Medical Alert Systems

Assistive Technology
Assistive technology is a broad term and may mean different things to different people but for our purposes we will define it as the following:

1. Devices or systems to help people who have no skilled medical needs manage their disabilities
2. Devices or systems that may also support disabilities with people who are receiving Medicare home care (durable home medical equipment)
3. Personal items or devices that make life easier for people with disabilities
4. Living environments that accommodate disability
5. Consultants, books and other advice
6. Home modification

As a general rule Medicare will reimburse 80% of the cost for rental or purchase of devices or systems that support disabilities due to a medical problem. Some items on the list provided below may also be included in Medicare's list of allowable durable medical equipment. Following is our list of devices in this category:

- Lifts
- Oxygen equipment
- Sensory Augmentation Devices
- Computer Usage Arrangements for the Disabled
- Wheelchairs and Scooters
- Other mobility related devices

Consultants, Books and Other Advice

There are numerous books available from bookstores and from online sources that give advice to caregivers in all areas of disability support. These sources often go beyond the issue of devices and equipment and deal with such things as meal preparation, menus, activities, music, and other social issues important to the disabled. Private and government consulting is also available. Check online or dial 211 or call the local area agency on aging for more help.

Home Modification

Many people with disabilities want to remain in their home as long as possible. Such things as narrow doorways that cannot accommodate wheelchairs, more than one living level, and inconvenient layout of the home may prevent a person from living there. In addition, disabled people often require rails, special bathroom facilities, and special dining accommodations as well. There are three options to modifying the home:

- Research can be done and materials procured to make the home more livable, and a family friend, or relative can pitch in and do the remodel.
- A contractor can be employed to do the necessary modifications.
- An attempt can be made to find a local company that specializes in full-package movement modification for the

disabled. These providers may be readily available in larger population areas.

In addition, help can be sought from the following community service providers:

- Local area agency on aging
- State department on aging
- State housing finance agency
- Department of public welfare
- Department of housing and community development
- Senior center Independent living center

The National Association of Home Builders and the AARP have teamed together to form the Certified Aging-in-Place Specialist (CAPS) program. These people have been trained in the unique needs of the older adult population, aging-in-place home modifications, common remodeling projects, and solutions to common barriers. It may be possible to find a person in the desired area by going to http://www.nahb.org/or by calling the local home builders association and asking for someone certified in this area.

Medical Alert Systems, Tracking and Prevention Devices

This area of assistance focuses more on the use of devices that warn of problems with homebound people who are often without caregivers for certain periods of the day. This may include:

- 24-hour vital sign monitoring
- video surveillance
- emergency signaling systems (medical alert) or
- GPS locator devices for wandering care recipients.

These services are very popular and can be found in the Yellow Pages or on the internet at www.longtermcarelink.net.

6. Elder Law and Estate Planning Advisors

Many elderly rely entirely on family or other trusted individuals to help them. Whether it is physiological or psychological, as people grow older, they tend to grow more childlike. The dependence upon caregivers or family members makes an older person more vulnerable for abuse and financial exploitation. Legal arrangements and protective actions by family may be necessary to shield loved ones from abuse.

Making legal decisions about property, finances, power of attorney, and last rights are important tasks to complete in planning for long term care. Having legal documentation for your will, assets, and whom you designate to be responsible for your welfare can avoid family disputes, abuse of your needs and finances, and conserve your assets for your care.

Elder Law Attorney
Elder law attorneys specialize in legal issues affecting the elderly. They are expert in Medicare and Medicaid programs and working with the elderly in assisting them and their families with all aspects of planning and implementing necessary legal documents.

Qualified legal help is available from most elder law attorneys to help individuals in applying for and accelerating payments for Medicaid. An elder law attorney can also help with disputes with Medicaid. Likewise attorneys who specialize in Medicare can help with disability claims. Sometimes this help is the only way claims are ever granted.

Below is a partial list of what an elder law attorney might do:

- Preservation or transfer of assets seeking to avoid spousal impoverishment when a spouse enters a nursing home
- Medicaid qualification and application and Medicaid planning strategies
- Medicare claims and appeals
- Social security and disability claims and appeals

- Disability planning, including use of durable powers of attorney, living trusts and living wills
- Help with financial management and health care decisions; and other means of delegating management and decision-making to another in case of incompetence or incapacity
- Probate
- Administration and management of trusts and estates
- Long term care placements in nursing homes and assisted living
- Nursing home issues with patients' rights and nursing home quality
- Elder abuse and fraud recovery cases

Estate Planning Attorney
The estate planning attorney provides information and legal advice for preparing your properties and finances so they transfer in the most efficient manner to your heirs. This also includes tax planning to avoid such things as estate taxes, state inheritance taxes and capital gains taxes on properties or investments.

Most attorneys who specialize in elder law, also provide estate planning advice.

An estate planning attorney will help you with the following:

- Give tax advice pertaining to estate issues
- Perform probate services
- Draw up wills and trusts
- Design powers of attorney and other consent documents
- Design special trusts or partnership programs to save estate or gift taxes
- Design charitable gifting programs
- Design strategies to transfer business ownership with death or disability
- Design programs to pay for estate taxes

Durable Power of Attorney
Many people do not know the difference between a general and a durable power of attorney. A general power of attorney is a document by which you appoint a person to act as your agent.

Agents are authorized to make decisions for you, sign legal documents, etc. Many people are unaware that a <u>General</u> Power of Attorney is revoked when the person granting that power becomes incompetent for incapacitated. It is the <u>"Durable"</u> Power of Attorney that allows for an agent to continue making decisions on your behalf no matter what happens to you.

A responsible adult child of an aging parent would be given a "durable power of attorney" to act on behalf of the parent. This provides broader authority than just adding the child's name to bank accounts and documents. Another form of durable power of attorney called a "springing power of attorney" allows for a more restrictive use of the power to act on your behalf.

Living Will and Advance Directives
A living will is your declaration made as to what actions you want taken in keeping you alive when you are in a vegetative state or there is no hope for recovery. You may want little or no medical intervention or life prolonging action. You set the limits in your will. You should entrust your living will to a person who knows your wishes and will ensure that they are observed.

CELA
A Certified Elder Law Attorney (CELA) has studied the legal needs of elders, the rules of Medicaid and Medicare and handled a requisite number of pertinent cases in order to receive that designation. This experience will make this person more informed about elder care issues.

You can find an Elder Law Attorney in your area on <u>www.longtermcarelink.net</u>.

Costs for Legal Help
Elder law and estate planning attorney costs are paid for out of private funds. Fees vary and are usually charged by hourly service.

State Legal Services
Most state bar associations have attorney referral programs or can direct you to an attorney referral program. There are also programs to provide some free legal service for people with low income. .

7. Elder Mediation Services

What Is Elder Mediation?

It is amazing how quickly formerly cordial relationships between family members will sour when the family has to deal with care of elderly parents or inheritance at their death. Sometimes the consequence of dealing with the final years of elderly parents can break families apart and create long lasting animosity.

Elder mediation is a promising new tool to help families heal broken relations, solve difficult issues arising from dealing with elderly parents, or prevent misunderstandings or problems from happening in the first place.

Mediation has been around for a long time, but only recently is it being applied to solving problems with elder care. The term "elder mediation" is still not widely used and someone seeking services in this area would most likely contact a "family mediator." Elder mediation is a rapidly growing specialization in the area of family mediation.

A mediator is a neutral third party who typically has no relationship with the family members who are in dispute or disagreement. The mediator brings the disputing people together, sits them down in the same room, and causes them to talk to each other. The mediator's role is to negotiate a resolution to the problem that is causing the disagreement. The mediator does not dictate or make decisions for the disputing parties but finds ways to facilitate communication between them. The goal of mediation is to produce a written agreement that all parties will abide by.

It is amazing how little some families communicate with each other. Perhaps when they grew up together, they were not accustomed to coming together as parents and children and working out problems. Now that children are older and taking care of parents, they don't have this family council strategy to rely on.

It may seem unnatural to them. But that is often exactly what is needed, especially in situations where, perhaps, one child is caring for the parents and the others are left out of the loop.

Children all have a common bond to their parents, and as a result a common obligation or responsibility to each other. When disagreements arise, suspicions begin to grow. Suspicions or distrust often lead to anger and the anger often leads to severing the channels of communication between family members.

This breaking up of ties can occur between parent and child or between siblings or between all of them. It is often at this point that a neutral third party can come in and repair the damage that has been done and help correct the problems that have come about because of the disagreement. A mediator experienced in elder mediation is a perfect choice for solving disagreements due to issues with the elderly.

Companies specializing in dispute resolution can also provide elder mediation services if a member of the firm specializes in this area. These companies, however, are more likely to serve deep-pocketed corporate clients, and their fees might be prohibitive. Such firms may charge an upfront administrative fee of $500 or more before they will even get to a session. Then they may charge $200 or more an hour for their services in a formal mediation. Finally they will charge an additional fee for writing up a final agreement.

Independent mediators may be individuals who have training in mediation and who specialize in specific areas of mediation. These are the people most likely to be of help to families needing elder mediation. Some of these people may actually specialize in elder mediation, and they are likely to have a background as a care manager, a social worker, a gerontologist, or a psychologist.

Those who specialize in elder mediation are most likely to have a background dealing with issues with the elderly. Others of these providers may be able to help with elder mediation, but their specialty may be broader, and they will typically present themselves as being family mediators.

Depending on their reputation and their effectiveness, independent mediators may charge anywhere from $50 per hour to $150 per hour. They may charge additional fees to formalize and make copies of the final agreement.

Disagreements Suitable for Elder Mediation

Elder mediation is a brand-new field and is still finding its roots, but those active in this area have identified the following issues with older people that can lead to disagreement, conflict or dispute:

- parental living arrangements
- health and personal care (such as driving ability)
- provisions in the case of terminal illness,
- home upkeep and repair
- financial concerns
- nursing home care
- trust and estate issues
- guardianship
- power of attorney
- relationships between parents, grandparents and grandchildren

We can talk about principles and ideas all day, but one cannot fully realize the vision of how mediation can help unless one encounters actual examples where it would apply.

Here is one example:

Sally and Jane are taking care of their aging parents who are living in their own home but need special help with bathing, dressing, and preparing their meals. Sally and Jane have their own families and both are employed. They trade off spending their evenings with their parents and one of them has gone to part-time employment in order to help the parents in the morning.

Their parents renovated the family home many years ago and created an apartment in the basement in order to produce rental income in their old age. They also have an additional rental property that provides further additional income.

Their married son -- Sally and Jane's brother -- with his wife and two teenage children are living in the basement apartment and paying no rent. He is out of work and has had difficulty in the past remaining employed. He does not help with the care of his parents and the parents are actually using most of their income to support him. Sally and Jane are angry. They need their parents to understand how they feel about the situation.

A mediator is the perfect solution for solving this problem.

Finding an Elder Mediator
Most mediators have training and experience in the area that they are working. Most can produce evidence of certification. The number of cases processed and the background of the person offering this service is an important consideration in the selection. Here are some suggestions for finding this service:

- Yellow Pages, look under "mediation services"
- Internet search, try some of the following web sites:
  http://www.searchamediator.com/
  http://www.mediate.com
  www.longtermcarelink.net
- Contact the local area agency on aging
- Contact your state bar association
- Contact a local university or college and asked to speak to the department that provides mediation training and ask for a referral.
- Contact a care manager: many care managers may also be mediators or may know an elder mediator.

8. Guardianship and Trust Administration

Guardianship

According to the American Bar Association Commission on Law and Aging, guardianship and conservatorship involve the following:

"Guardianship or Conservatorship is the legal tool of last resort for decision-making and management of your affairs."

A guardian is usually court-appointed to manage the property and/or personal affairs of persons who are not capable to do so for themselves. Conservatorship typically involves management of just one's assets without control over the person. The court can limit the guardian's authority to specific areas of need or give unlimited power to the guardian..

People need a guardian when they cannot make decisions themselves and serious harm may come to them. In its most basic form, guardianship of person encompasses the job of making decisions for a person who has been legally declared incapacitated, incompetent or legally disabled.

If you already have an agent or family member under a durable power of attorney or under a health care advance directive, the court will normally determine that the agent's or family member's authority shall continue to function.

Because of the critical nature of the relationships among those involved - the family, the individual protected person and the guardian, the National Guardianship Association, Inc. (NGA) certifies guardians and encourages them to adopt a specific code of ethics. It provides its members with education and training and the opportunity to set a national agenda to ensure standards of excellence.

Trust Administration and Management

A trust is a legal document that "entrusts" property to a trustee to manage that property for a person or persons whom the maker of the trust wants to benefit. In most cases, the maker of a trust is creating a benefit for a loved one that will be distributed after his or her death. Trusts usually involve very specific and detailed instructions on how a trustee is to carry out the duty of managing or distributing the property on behalf of a beneficiary. A trustee can be a bank, an attorney, an individual, or a trust company.

A trustee will manage investments, keep records, manage assets, and prepare court accountings -- paying bills and (depending on the nature of the trust) medical expenses, charitable gifts, inheritances or other distributions of income and principal.

A trust relationship is also created in a will when the maker of the will specifies an entity to be an executor or personal representative of the estate. This person or company then becomes a trustee for the deceased individual who made the will. The responsibilities of an executor in settling the estate of a deceased person include collecting debts, settling claims for debt and taxes, accounting for assets to the courts, and distributing wealth to beneficiaries.

A third party trust officer such as a bank, attorney or trust company may also assume the role of a guardian for a minor child, distributing assets in a prearranged manner when the child becomes an adult. Or the trust officer may also act on behalf of a developmentally disabled or mentally retarded person distributing assets under a special needs trust.

Trusts are most often used with estate planning. The purpose of estate planning is to minimize the cost and streamline the process of distributing assets to the next generation. Here are some of the more common reasons people create trusts in estate planning:

- To avoid probate
- To minimize or eliminate estate taxes
- To create life insurance trusts
- To avoid capital gains taxes on the sale of property
- To create an annuity income through charitable gifting
- To receive a charitable gifting income tax deduction
- To manage assets on behalf of a minor or someone who cannot handle his or her own affairs

Trust companies are valuable partners in the management of trusts and in the process of estate planning. These companies, for a small fee, will manage and invest assets, maintain escrow accounts, hold property pending an exchange sale, provide life insurance and income annuities, and provide safekeeping of valuables.

Many people who create trusts or wills or both will designate a trust company or bank to be a trustee for their property instead of using a member of the family or close friend to do this. The reason is that, all too often, assets are mismanaged or even stolen by family members or friends. Using a trust company that has a legally mandated, public fiduciary responsibility avoids this problem. Find a trust administration specialist in your area on www.longtermcarelink.net

9. Financial Services Specialists

Now is the time to review your insurance policies, bank accounts, retirement accounts, annuities, bonds, and any other financial documents or plans that you have set up.

Insurance Specialists
Specialists in insurance have extensive knowledge in the products they offer and can give you the information you need for planning long term care.

Types of insurance specialists for long term care planning.

- Life insurance
- Long term care insurance
- Medicare Advantage, supplement and drug plan specialists
- Annuities

There are many reputable companies that provide these products. We advise you do some research, get referrals from friends that are satisfied with their agent and his or her products.

Financial Advisor
A financial planner or advisor, who works with the elderly, is going to understand how to manage assets for that age group. This person will also understand how to use assets and income when there is a need for long term care.

A financial adviser will work closely with an estate planning or elder law attorney to make sure all arrangements for the estate, for disability, for loss of capacity, for medical treatment, and for long term care are covered.

An elder financial adviser is also likely to work with a team of other eldercare providers or advisers such as care managers, pre-need funeral planners, long term care insurance specialists, reverse mortgage specialists and home health providers.

Services covered by a financial advisor:

- Investment advice
- Income tax
- Retirement planning
- Small business
- Protection and insurance
- Estate planning
- Saving for education
- Asset allocation
- General financial planning

You can locate more information on insurance and financial planning products and find specialists in your area on www.longtermcarelink.net.

10. Reverse Mortgage Specialist

With most people, their home is their biggest investment. This one investment can provide the money you may need for your long term care planning. In Step 2, Reverse Mortgages were discussed as an option for paying for long term care services, home repairs or alterations or just having money for wanted items.

When you have decided to obtain a reverse mortgage, you then must determine what type of loan to use. The U.S. Department of Housing and Urban Development's popular home-equity conversion mortgage (HECM) is insured by the federal government. The amount of loan you can obtain with HECM is determined by the FHA lending limit in your area. If you own a high-value house, you may be better off with a loan from Fannie Mae or from a private lender.

Because reverse mortgages may be confusing, you are required to meet with a counselor before you can apply and to be sure you understand the pros and cons as well as how the reverse mortgage works. A reverse mortgage is a major decision and the time spent with the counselor is well worth your peace of mind for your future.

A reverse mortgage specialist works in conjunction with a lending company. Some may be under contract with one company and others may offer services of multiple lending companies. A specialist usually only sells reverse mortgages and is expert in the rules and qualifications. A specialist will help you find the right mortgage for your needs and, set up your counseling appointment and complete the appraisal and necessary documents.

You can locate more information on Reverse Mortgages and find specialists in your area on www.longtermcarelink.net

11. Seniors Relocation and Real Estate Specialists

As people age, they often become overly attached to their homes and even though there may be compelling reasons to find other living arrangements, these folks will go to extreme lengths to remain in their homes.

Notwithstanding the affection for their dwellings, there is oftentimes undeniable pressure for seniors to move out and into different living arrangements. Consider the following:

- The challenge of maintaining a yard and providing upkeep has become too great.
- There is a need for long term care that can't be handled in the home.
- The older person needs supervision that can't be provided in the home.
- The neighborhood has deteriorated and safety is a concern.
- There is a desire to be near children or grandchildren (70% of those 65+ live within 1 hour of a child).
- The home cannot accommodate disability needs.
- There is a need to avoid climbing stairs.
- Assets are tied up in the home and cash is needed through selling the property.
- Driving is no longer possible and available local transportation is not adequate.
- There is a desire for a warmer climate, a yearning for new vistas or a need for challenging new experiences.

Typically, the thought of giving up their residences, finding new accommodations, downsizing personal possessions and executing the move can seem overwhelming to many older people.

Perhaps another obstacle for many seniors, contemplating a move, is the lack of support or help from family members. In fact, some seniors have no children. For others, the children are living far away or are extremely busy with their jobs or their own families. And in some cases -- because people are living so long -- the children are elderly as well and find it difficult to help with the move.

This overwhelming pressure and stress relating to moving can often result in gridlock -- a failure to make any decision at all.

Because many elderly people face such a daunting task with moving, a growing number of seniors' relocation specialists are stepping forward to provide assistance. These individuals or companies provide or arrange for the following services:

- advice and counseling,
- help with finding new accommodations,
- downsizing possessions through personal, caring assistance with discarding, donating or arranging estate sales,
- selling the existing property,
- organizing, arranging and scheduling the move,
- unpacking at the new location and removing boxes and other debris,
- setting up and arranging furniture.

And it isn't just the elderly person, contemplating a move, who is hiring these specialists. Active senior communities, independent living facilities, nursing homes and assisted living often retain a relocation specialist to provide advice and arrange services to help seniors with a move. Family members of seniors have also found it more convenient to hire a specialist to help their loved ones with relocation.

So who are these companies or individuals who provide seniors relocation and real estate services?

Seniors Real Estate Specialists
A Seniors Real Estate Specialist (SRES) is a real estate agent who specializes in helping the elderly transition to a new location. The specialist has been trained to recognize the special needs of seniors and understand the various living arrangements available to older people. Most of these specialists concentrate on selling the property and do not directly provide relocation services but they will arrange for companies or individuals or advisors who can provide these other services.

Senior Move Managers

A Senior Move Manager is a member of the National Association of Senior Move Managers. These people often have a background in social work or case management and have experience working with the elderly. As such, they understand the needs and desires of seniors. Senior Move Managers can provide or arrange for any needed service such as counseling and advice, selling property, downsizing or relocating their clients.

Moving Companies

Many independent moving companies recognize the special needs of seniors and they will provide moving services, storage and other specialized programs for this unique group of customers. These companies will often work together with senior advisors and relocation specialists.

Specialists with Developers or Senior Communities

Active senior community developers, senior residences and care facilities have recognized that providing relocation services will help their clients or residents transition more quickly into the new living arrangements. This not only relieves the stress on the seniors but also results in less cost to the providers who might be holding open properties or rooms for a long period of time due to the difficulty of selling the old residence and relocating.

Professional Organizers

Professional organizers -- many of whom are members of the National Association of Professional Organizers -- have found a unique niche in helping people reduce clutter in their homes or provide a more efficient office or living environment. Because of extensive experience in reducing personal possessions, a professional organizer can be particularly useful in helping to downsize in anticipation of a move.

Professional or Geriatric Care Managers

Most care managers help people, needing long term care, to find appropriate living arrangements. A natural outgrowth of finding new accommodations has resulted in many care managers specializing in relocation services as part of what they do.

12. Hospice Care Providers

Some people are content to leave decisions regarding their death in the hands of others. By doing so, they may expose themselves to unnecessary and futile treatments to prolong their life. They may also experience numerous visits to the emergency room in the last stages of their life. This dependency on others often results in great stress to family members, when elders lose their capacity and have not made their last wishes known. Family is often forced to make decisions about life support and treatment without knowing whether their loved one would have wanted these interventions.

Adding a knowledge of hospice care to your plan provides assurance your last days or those of a loved one will be spent where and how you want.

There are companies that specialize only in hospice care. Or it is often the case that home health agencies also offer hospice. Hospice provides a team of specialists that work under your physician's orders to provide every aspect of care.

This could include:

- Hospice case manager
- Nurse
- Physical therapist
- Dietician
- Social worker
- Bereavement counselors

Hospice is generally used for cancer patients because it is often easy to determine in advance whether a person will survive or not. If the cancer is not cured and continues to spread, death is usually inevitable. Whether that occurs in a matter of weeks or months is not important to the doctor prescribing hospice. The only requirement is the doctor must have a reasonable expectation that his patient cannot survive beyond six months. Sometimes hospice patients can receive care for years before they succumb.

For other medical conditions, hospice may be just as appropriate, but oftentimes the family fails to inquire or the family doctor simply doesn't consider it. Hospice should be considered for such conditions as congestive heart failure, advanced diabetes, advanced lung disease, advanced autoimmune disorders, advanced kidney disease and so on. Even in the absence of any medical condition, a person can still qualify for hospice if he or she is deteriorating rapidly and overall health is declining.

Another condition often overlooked for hospice is advanced dementia or Alzheimer's disease. Families often wait until a loved one starts shutting down before hospice is ordered. Or sometimes hospice is not even considered for Alzheimer's because doctors are so used to using this care only for cancer.

If a loved one is not improving, family should always ask or even press for hospice. Remember not to wait until close to the end but order hospice at an earlier stage since it will help provide the transition to the death of a loved one in a more dignified way.

Home Telehospice
A new service is being introduced into the hospice care program – home telehospice. It provides 24 hour nursing support for the caregiver without the nurse being physically in the home. Videophones installed in the home enables a caregiver to call with questions or to get instructions from a nurse in doing care procedures and monitoring a hospice patient.

The nurse or other medical persons can view the patient and determine what needs to be done. They can then instruct the caregiver. This service relieves questions and concerns that often pop up late at night without one of the hospice staff traveling to the home. Under most conditions, Medicare will cover home telehospice. As with telehealth, this service is more suitable for rural areas where driving long distances to make visits is difficult or impossible.

You can locate Hospice services in your local phone book, online searches under hospice, or locate a company in your area on www.longtermcarelink.net

13. PrePlanning, PreNeed Funeral Providers

A funeral director or employee trained in preplanned arrangements can help you and your family make the decisions and preparations for future funeral and burial needs.

Death often places unanticipated burdens on the family both emotionally and financially. Prearranging removes that burden from family. Privately or with family members, you meet with the preplanning director and arrange all or part of the burial and funeral services. This is put into a contract ready to use at a later date.

Prefunding the funeral also relieves the financial burden from your survivors. These are paid by putting money into a special irrevocable trust fund, escrow account or insurance policy. At the time of death, the funds are paid to the funeral director.

Following are some advantages of preplanning:

- It provides peace of mind knowing these arrangements have been made in advance.
- It avoids the burden on family members to make decisions when they are most vulnerable to manipulation.
- It helps the family to avoid taking loans, arranging finance plans, raiding savings, or selling assets to pay for a funeral and burial.
- It guarantees (for many contracts) that if products and services currently purchased are not available in the future, equivalent substitutes will be provided at no additional cost. It locks in guaranteed prices (with some contracts) forever.
- It allows for inflation in future costs (for those contracts that do not guarantee prices) by investing money in an interest-bearing account or buying life insurance that increases in value over time.

Most funeral homes have a preplanning director. Check with local facilities. To find out more about preplanning or locate a director go to www.longtermcarelink.net

STEP 4

Creating a Personal Care Plan and Choosing a Care Coordinator

Success is assured through a written plan; accepted by all parties involved.

The previous three steps in this book have given you a wealth of information about long term care. It is important for you to have an understanding of care systems and the resources you can turn to when the need arises. However, knowledge of long term care services is not enough. You must take some action now to prepare for the day when you will need to deal with eldercare for your loved ones or for yourself.

This final fourth step in the planning process is designed to help you make a care plan. If you follow the instructions in this section and prepare a plan for you or a loved one, the challenge of dealing with long term care will unfold for you in a more manageable manner. You will experience less stress, have fewer costs, require less time committed and have fewer family conflicts.

If the care plan is for you and you are currently healthy and able to handle your own affairs, then only you or you with your spouse will create your personal plan. This is about you, your preparation and wishes in the event of needing long term care.

If you are the child or other family member, a trusted friend or an adviser who is reading this book to understand how to help a loved one or client deal with impending long term care, then you will be helping that person prepare a plan for himself or herself.

This last step is divided into two parts. Part I will introduce how this book becomes your single-source planning reference and introduces you to the process of creating a plan and documenting all the information that will be needed. You will complete a survey form that will help you see what resources you already have and what additional information, financial products and documents you need to acquire.

Choosing a care coordinator and holding a planning and agreement meeting with all family or friends that will be involved will be your final step.

Part II contains the following forms:

1. "Checklist for Making a Long Term Care Plan"
2. "Care Planning Survey"
3. "Personal Long Term Care Plan"
4. "Care Planning Agreement"

These planning forms are designed for you to record all necessary important information for your long term care plan. Part II pages are yellow in color in order to identify that this section of the book is the written part of the care plan.

There is also a duplicate perforated copy of the long term care planning checklist at the very back of the book. Please remove this and use it as you go through Part I. There is a permanent copy of this checklist in Part II for your record as well.

A perforated copy of the care planning agreement is also at the end of the book on page 159. Remove this and write on it the same information found in the agreement that is in the book. Make copies of this form for every person attending your planning and agreement meeting who will be involved in the long term care plan.

PART I – OVERVIEW OF THE LONG TERM CARE PLANNING PROCESS

<u>With the information in this book in hand, you are ready to create a long term care plan. Please remove the perforated copy of the checklist on page 161 to aid you as you go through Part I.</u>

There are basically two planning scenarios for two different categories of people who need long term care planning.

The first of these planning scenarios involves older individuals who are currently receiving long term care or for whom the need for care is imminent. Most of these individuals are not prepared financially to pay the cost of care. Most have also neglected to involve family or other persons close to them in dealing with the possibility that long term care might be needed. Family and friends are often caught unaware and are often forced to work in a crisis mode trying to solve the problems associated with providing care for their loved one.

With these people already receiving care, some of the elements of planning are missing, but a carefully designed plan can still solve a lot of problems and relieve a lot of stress. Our care planning process can be followed step-by-step for this group but the personal long term care plan that results will constantly be changing as the need for care evolves.

Consider the following example of a care plan for someone needing immediate care:
Shelley has been watching out for and helping her mother since her father died of a sudden heart attack a year ago. Shelley's mother is 77 and her husband, Shelley's father, was a veteran of Korea. Her mother has arthritis and has difficulty bathing, dressing and moving around and she is also exhibiting early signs of dementia.

Mother makes $800 a month in Social Security, has $2,000 in savings and owns her own home. She has substantial consumer debt that she is burdened with and she cannot make ends meet. Shelley has been helping her meet her obligations. Mother also takes

117

advantage of the low income utilities programs and other government support to help the elderly poor.

A good friend and neighbor comes in the morning to help mother get dressed and to fix her breakfast and Meals on Wheels comes at noon to leave her lunch. Shelley comes by in the late afternoon, after work, and fixes her mother dinner, helps her get a bath if necessary and gets her ready for bed. Shelley spends her entire weekends with her mother. Shelley has no husband or children but she also has no life of her own because of the care of her mother.

Her brothers and sisters, who also live in the area, are perfectly happy with this arrangement because they have their own families and they think everything is under control. They have made no offers to help, other than to take mom shopping or to the doctor. However, they always seem to have plenty of advice for Shelley. Shelley feels trapped.

Sheliey attends a caregiving presentation during her lunch break at work and obtains a copy of our book "The 4 Steps of Long Term Care Planning." After reading the book, she realizes she has many more options than she thought and she feels empowered to take better control of the caregiving morass she has fallen into.

By following our checklist, she investigates all of the caregiving options available to her. She completes the worksheet section of the book. She next consults with a financial planner and an elder law attorney to understand funding and legal issues.

Her next step is to arrange a meeting between her, her mother and her brothers and sisters.

Mother is absolutely adamant about staying in her home as long as she can, and because her family loves her, they want to respect her wishes as far as humanly possible.

Shelley has uncovered the following solutions for care:

1. As a result of reading our book, Shelley discovered the value of using a care manager. Shelley hired a care manager to do an assessment of her mother and the care manager had a number of valuable recommendations, including the involvement of other family members. The care manager, who is a nurse, also feels that mother's arthritis could be treated more adequately to provide some improvement. She also suspects the mild dementia is probably due to poor nutrition, lack of stimulation and depression and is not an organic condition. The care manager has suggested a geriatrician for Shelley's mother, who has an excellent reputation for diagnosing and treating and improving health conditions in the elderly.

2. Because Shelley's father was a veteran, her mother can get an additional $976 a month from VA to cover home care costs.

3. Her mother can qualify for a reverse mortgage to pay off the debt and turn remaining funds into an additional lifetime income to allow her to stay in the home.

4. Someone needs to have power of attorney and there must be a plan in place with what to do with the house in case mother can no longer live at home and must go to a facility. The attorney and financial planner have offered some good suggestions.

Because of her demanding schedule as caregiver and working full time, Shelley needs help from her family in arranging for these solutions and in giving her the additional support she needs as a caregiver. She has a long talk with her older brother and helps him understand the situation and he agrees to call a family meeting. He also agrees to discuss the situation with other family members and to come away with an agreement between them all on how to support their mother in the home and help Shelley as the caregiver.

The family meets together and the older brother--using our planning checklist as an agenda--goes over the entire scenario with the others, who up to this point have been content to let Shelley handle everything and really do not know all that is going on.

Agreements are made for members of the family to assume responsibilities for completing the solutions to the care plan. The older brother will be power of attorney and be responsible for the finances because he is a CPA. In addition, by understanding their sister's plight, other family members agree to help with the caregiving as well.

An agreement is drawn up and everyone is given a copy. The older brother has been designated as the care coordinator and he assumes ownership of the care planning book with the worksheet forms and the original care agreement. He also buys copies of the book for other members of the family because he wants them to understand all of the options available.

His ultimate responsibility is to make sure that all solutions and other options have been explored to provide the best care for their mother; and in addition, that everyone lives up to his or her promise made in the care agreement.

~~~~~~~~~~~~~~~~~~~~~~~~~~~

The second group that should be doing long term care planning is individuals who are currently healthy but want to plan for the day when they will need help. Ideally, planning prior to retirement is the best time because it affords the opportunity to prepare financially to pay the cost of long term care. If you are healthy and young enough, long term care insurance should be purchased. If this is not possible, then money should be put away in savings to cover the cost.

Some of our readers might be in their retirement years but still healthy and not needing care. These people should most definitely plan now and prepare their families or friends for helping them someday with the need for long term care. Even for this group, some financial preparation can be made to help pay the cost.

Consider the following examples to illustrate the planning process where people are healthy and currently don't need care:

Example #1--Planning after Retirement

Mary, age 75, is trying to prepare her son to avoid the mistakes she made with her husband Bill. Five years ago, Bill lost his ability to communicate due to early-onset Alzheimer's. He also suffered from heart disease and diabetes. As his caregiver, Mary was never quite sure she was making the right choices about his long term care and medical treatment. Eventually Bill needed life support and Mary agonized over how Bill really would have wanted his life to end, since they had never discussed it. Bill died last year. So many things were left undone regarding his care.

Mary has decided to plan for long term care and medical treatment before it happens. She has designated her son as her personal care coordinator. She has given him written instructions in the planning pages of our book regarding different care scenarios and how to prepare for caregiving. He also has copies of her will and trust as well as other legal care documents. Through our planning book, Mary has provided him an extensive source of long term care information as well as a list of her personal financial resources.

Mary has implemented the financial solutions to pay for her care. And finally, she has provided her son, in the book planning pages, a detailed list of government and private long term care service providers in her area. She has also given her son a copy of our book with all of the information pertaining to her financial records, her care plan and her legal arrangements.

By planning in advance for long term care, Mary has removed the guilt that loved ones feel in making care choices for her. She has researched and given direction on the types of care she desires, she has given direction and guidance to would-be caregivers and lastly she has planned for the means to pay for that care.

Example #2--Planning Prior to Retirement

Alice, age 56, and Frank, age 59, are the parents of three grown children. Their two oldest children live out of state. Their youngest, Andrea, is married with one child and lives about 40 miles away.

Alice is an educator and in 6 more years she will be eligible for a retirement pension. She has also managed to put away a small nest egg with the State 401(k) and in a tax sheltered annuity. Frank is self-employed and other than Social Security, he will have no other retirement income or savings.

Alice went through long term care with both of her parents. Her mother died 3 years ago and her father died 5 years ago. Alice was the only one of her brothers and sisters willing or able to care for her parents. Between trying to maintain a very demanding profession and provide care support to her single mother in the morning and evening and on weekends, it was all she could do to avoid a nervous breakdown. At the same time, her youngest daughter, Andrea, was a senior in high school and although, Andrea was mostly self-sufficient, Alice still feels the guilt of not being there for Andrea because of the burden in caring for her parents.

Alice's career also suffered as she was unable to attend continuing education courses to meet career ladder thresholds and she had to opt out of extra activities at school. Her principal was understanding but she wasn't sure about her standing with the rest of the staff and administration.

Alice has persuaded Frank to set up a long term care plan for themselves to avoid the mistakes made with her parents. They recently purchased long term care insurance policies that combined with their incomes will allow them to maintain their home and provide enough to pay for professional help to keep them in the home.

If for some reason they can't stay at home, the insurance will pay for institutional care as well. If one of them dies and the other goes to live with Andrea, the insurance will allow their daughter to oversee professional in-home care and respite care and not be tied down as her mother was with caregiving.

Alice and Frank want their children to have their house and they have set up a will and trust to provide for an orderly distribution. Alice has made a list of who-gets-what of her keepsakes and has listed the things she wants her grandchildren to remember their grandparents by. They have asked Andrea to be their personal care coordinator and have given her instructions, in the planning pages of our book, regarding care, financial resources, community resources and legal documents.

Alice and Frank place their information in our book and give the book to Andrea to help her carry out her future responsibility. They also buy a copy for themselves for the day when they will need this information as well.

Because Alice and Frank have put everything in order, they feel they will not be the burden on Andrea and her family that Alice's parents caused for her and her family.

Understand How This Book Becomes Your Care Plan

This book provides comprehensive information about long term care planning. The design also allows you to record personal information, agreements and directions on planning sheets at the back of the book.

Using the book as a single-source repository for information and directions makes it much easier for you or your care coordinator to carry out your wishes.

The following design features make this book a unique and outstanding resource for long term care planning:

1. The book is a comprehensive source of information about community, government and private long term care services.

2. The book provides a survey in order for the planner to determine what care resources are missing and what documents, services, products and decisions are necessary in designing a well-functioning plan.

3. The book is a repository for information about your personal resources, your planning documents, your financial products and your insurance; and it contains your written instructions for carrying out your personal long term care plan.

4. The book contains an agreement between all involved persons that spells out commitments from those persons for supporting your personal long term care plan.

Fill out the Care Planning Survey

In order to proceed with the actions necessary to complete a plan, you first need to fill out the "Care Planning Survey." This is found in the yellow-colored pages, beginning on page 143.

The information you gain from this exercise will help you to determine care preferences for you or a loved one and what legal, end-of-life and financial arrangements must be made.

Determining care preferences will allow you to decide whether you or the loved one wants to remain in the home, go to assisted living or make other living arrangements. You will also have a good idea of whether you want members of the family to be involved in the care, or if you want to pay for professional care.

If there are members of the family or close friends or even a care manager who are willing, you or your loved one can also decide who is to be the care coordinator.

The survey will also help you understand whether there is funding available to pay for professional care or whether government programs can help provide that care. You may even discover some avenues of funding that you didn't know existed. For example, the veterans benefit. You will also find out what legal arrangements have to be made.

As you fill out the survey, make note of items or services you want to gather more information about. Refer back to Steps 1 through 3 as needed to review this information.

Gather Information

Having completed the care planning survey, you can more readily see areas where you want to gather more information as well as identifying personal, financial and legal documents you need. Having all of this information will allow you to go out and investigate options available in your community. You may want to make some calls to different community services and make note of what is available. This is the time to visit assisted living facilities or care centers and talk with home health agencies about their services.

If there is no need for immediate care, you can identify the type of services you want but not necessarily who will provide them. If there is an immediate need for care, you can go a step further and start making arrangements.

Legal arrangements can be made anytime during the care planning process. At this point--where you are gathering information--you may only want to identify what needs to be done and whom you want to help you with the legal work. After you have had a planning meeting, perhaps someone in that meeting may take the assignment of arranging for legal documents.

Just remember this. You must make the legal arrangements while you or your loved one is still competent. If you wait too long, the alternatives to gaining control with an incompetence issue are vastly more difficult.

The next three topics below (next 3 items on your checklist) will aid you in gathering and organizing needed documents in preparation for filling out your "Personal Long Term Care Plan" worksheets.

Choose a Personal Care Coordinator

Choosing a Personal Care Coordinator to help with the creation, the implementation, and the directives of a long term care plan is the most vital part of the planning process. This person is not the caregiver. This person carries out the plan and supports the caregiver.

Here is why the care coordinator is so important. If a caregiver is a family member, that person is almost always thrust into his or her role without preparation. The caregiver typically becomes enmeshed in making decisions for medical care, arranging doctor visits or hospital stays and in providing services and companionship for the care recipient. As such, the caregiver becomes distracted from arranging family support, finding resources or committing to counseling and training. The caregiver needs the support and direction that the Care Coordinator gives.

The Personal Care Coordinator becomes the advocate and guide in making sure all of the pieces of the puzzle fit together. A coordinator can be a child, a close friend, a sibling, a trusted advisor, a professional social worker, a counselor or a care manager. He or she has agreed to help make arrangements and to see that the written care agreement is being followed.

Below are some of the activities a Personal Care Coordinator might perform. The duties and the role the coordinator will play are spelled out in written instructions contained in the back of this book and created by you. Here are some sample directions.

- Make sure an assessment of the care recipient is made and a plan of care is designed.
- Become familiar with the community resources and planning strategies and help the caregiver use them.
- Make sure the caregiver receives counseling and training.
- If applicable, organize a family council and solicit caregiving commitments.
- Act as an advocate for the caregiver and make sure people honor their commitments.
- Help with transportation, arrangement of meals and visits from formal caregivers.
- Help with financial decisions if needed.
- Maintain copies of legal documents and make sure they are up-to-date.
- Accompany the caregiver on meetings with government agencies and provide advice with decisions that have to be made.
- Contact appropriate professional planners to advise about and implement financial strategies.
- Make sure that professional care providers are competent and that all professional options have been explored.
- Maintain copies of financial preparations to pay for care and help with putting them into effect.
- Make sure the written personal care plan is followed.

Identify Needed Legal and End-of-Life Arrangements

All legal documents must be researched, written and signed while one is mentally competent. Do not wait for the onset of illness or take a chance that a stroke or other physical trauma will render you or your loved one incompetent to handle affairs. If you wish, some of the legal documents can be done up by you and signed by the appropriate signatories.

We recommend you use an attorney to complete your documents. Elder law attorneys or estate planning attorneys specialize in preparing the types of documents for your long term care plan.

Gather all legal documents, titles, deeds, etc. and record information about each one on the form provided in the planning section--yellow colored pages--in this book. Record who--if anyone--has a copy of the documents and where the originals are kept. Be sure that the care coordinator has a copy of everything.

Will
Upon death you have a will whether you want one or not. State intestate laws prescribe the method in which property of the deceased owner passes to his heirs. If a person is satisfied with these rules, he needs no personal will. If he wants a different distribution of property, then he must devise a personal will which takes precedence over intestate rules.

Your state law may allow you to draw up a "holographic" will—a document all in the handwriting of and signed by the creator. In those states that recognize it, this is considered a legal document.

Or you may wish to create a formal will with an attorney. This is because if there are assets or intentions that are not clearly defined, it could cause all kinds of unforeseen problems for your heirs or loved ones. You may end up disinheriting someone by doing it yourself and creating the exact opposite of what you intended.

Living Will
A living will provides guidance about end-of-life such as whether or not you want ventilation, hydration or a feeding tube. A person can also use the document to reject other life-prolonging measures. In some States, the document takes effect only if the patient is expected

to die within six months or is in a persistent vegetative state and is unable to communicate to health care providers. Someone suffering from an accident or acute illness will be treated without regard to a living will.

If the patient can communicate, the document has no effect. Also the document can be revoked at any time and it is not binding on the patient.

In some states, you can also create a power of attorney for health care which can spell out in more detail the decisions for your care that can be made when you become incompetent. Or you can give a blank-card health care power of attorney which allows your agent to make any medical decision or medical financial decision for you.

The Physicians Orders For Life Sustaining Treatment (POLST)
A POLST form is a physician's order that records your wishes for resuscitation, use of antibiotics, artificially administered fluids and nutrition. You will need to speak to your physician about filling out this form and what directives you want for care.

Durable Power of Attorney
As stated in the section under "Elder Law Advice", you need a durable power of attorney to allow your personal care coordinator to function in your behalf when you become incapacitated in any way. It is very important for the correct documents to be drawn and signed when making your long term care plan.

Some of us are careful not to have a durable power of attorney in force while we can handle our affairs. There is a special kind of durable power of attorney called a "Springing Power of Attorney" which is more appropriate for this purpose.

Estate Planning -Trusts
There are countless types of trusts created for myriads of different situations but the most common trust, useful to most of us, is the "living" or "inter vivo" trust. The purpose of this trust is to avoid the cost, public disclosure and the potentially lengthy process of probate. If you have trusts, check with your estate planner or legal council to be sure they are set up correctly to transfer assets or provide instructions for taking care of your beneficiaries.

Who-Gets-What-List
Generally a will specifies the disposition of specific assets and such lists are incorporated into it. But, often the disposition of items with little intrinsic or economic value but immense sentimental or historical value is just as important if not more important to most us. These are such things as personal histories, achievement awards, genealogies, favorite ceramics, handicrafts, heirlooms, special furniture, pictures, collections, etc.

It is important to make a list of who-gets-what of the "special" belongings and update it regularly. Sometimes in the haste and confusion of arranging long term care, "treasures" end up in the trash or at the local thrift store. Or even more likely, they end up in the wrong hands. The improper distribution of assets can sometimes cause bad feelings or infighting between family members. This contention has even broken apart families.

Usually state law does not require such lists to be attached to the will and the list may not even require the help of a lawyer if there is no will. Giving copies of the list to the recipients should be sufficient enough intent for family members to respect final wishes. But, if you personally are doing the planning and are concerned about legal respect for your wishes, you can create the list in your own handwriting and sign it.

End-of-Life Services
Care recipients remaining in their own home or a family member's home, may have hospice attend to their last needs. Remember that generally Medicare pays for hospice, and the expert care from this service benefits everyone involved.

If a terminal patient is in a hospital or care facility, he or she can return home with hospice service. This provides an end-of-life experience in a more preferable setting.

Another end-of-life service that you can set up now is preplanned funeral arrangements. You or your family can visit your designated funeral home now and make all the arrangements needed for future services. Payment can also be prepaid, which relieves family of that financial burden.

Identify Financial, Government and Provider Resources

Bank Checking and Savings Information

List checking and savings accounts in the personal planning forms section of this book. Put account and PIN numbers if you feel safe in doing so. Eventually the Care Coordinator will need to have this information. Keep this list updated as time goes on.

List qualified tax deferred savings accounts such as an IRA, 401(k), TSA, 403(b), 457, SEPP, SIMPLE or 401(a). If you are creating this list prior to retirement you must continue to update the information after retirement and as you grow older.

If you want to designate funds from certain accounts to be spent for specific things, put those instructions on the planning sheets.

Life Insurance Policies

List all life insurance policies in the appropriate forms section. Record the policy numbers and contact information. If you have the name of the Insurance agent who sold the policy, add that as well.

Health Insurance or Advantage Plan

List health insurance policies, supplemental insurance or Advantage Plan policies. Put whom to contact about questions on these policies.

Medicare Prescription Drug Plan Insurance (if applicable)

List information about Medicare PDP insurance

Long Term Care Insurance

If there is long term care insurance, list the policy number and contact information. Now would be a good time to review the policy to be sure you understand what it will cover and how much.

Annuities and Trusts

If there are deferred annuities or special trust accounts, you should list them as well. Put pertinent information to allow the care coordinator to have access to the documents.

Other Assets

Continue to update this list as you get closer to needing care.

Monthly, Quarterly or Annual Income
Record income and the source, such as Social Security, retirement investment income, dividends, pension income, annuity income, rental property income, etc. If you're doing this planning prior to retirement you'll have to change this information after retirement.

Real Estate
The value of your home or other properties should be listed in case they need to be sold to pay for care. (Remember, a reverse mortgage may also help with financial needs) Keep the value updated.

Government and Community Services
Here is where your research pays off. You may want the care coordinator to fill this out with you as he or she will need this information as well. You will want a list of government services, what they can provide, with contact information ready, in place, for when needed.

Take time to call or visit community senior centers, area agencies on aging or other community services to see what is available. Books on tape, companionship services, and home-delivered meals are some services you may want to note for future reference.

Professional Services
Step 3 gave you an overview of long term care professionals and why they are a necessary part of a long term care plan.

If you or a loved one has chosen to stay at home or in the home of a family member, you will be looking at home care, both informal and formal. You may also need home maintenance and chore services or medical equipment or alert systems.

If the plan is for an assisted living arrangement, make note of those care services and what may be needed to supplement the services for future care. For instance, you can have a home care provider come into assisted living if you choose.

Review the services of a professional care manager. This person may offer the greatest help and support for you and the designated care coordinator. When the time comes that an extensive medical needs' plan of care is imminent, the professional care manager can make educated decisions without emotional involvement.

This can remove the burden from the chosen family care coordinator who may be hesitant to make nursing home or hospice arrangements on your behalf or on behalf of a loved one. There is emotional stress and uncertainty in such decisions, even with outlined directions in the care plan.

If the caregiver is not a family member, you may want the services of a professional care manager to oversee hiring and coordinating help with the care. She would work under the direction of the designated care coordinator.

Remember, the care coordinator and caregiver should not be the same person, especially if they are both family. The Care Coordinator needs to support and provide resources for the caregiver. It is extremely difficult for the caregiver and the coordinator to wear the same hat.

Family Mediator
If there is difficulty with involved family members or others agreeing on a plan of care, then use an elder or family mediator. Some professional care managers are also mediators.

With the consent of everyone involved, you can secure the services of a mediator when holding the care planning meeting. It is surprising how many families are torn apart because of feelings and jealousy that happen with a parent's long term care. The mediator will help each person express his or her feelings and concerns and resolve any conflicts.

Record the types and names of the professional services you may want to use on the care planning sheets in this book beginning on page 147.

Complete "Personal Long Term Care Plan" Worksheets

This is the focus of the entire planning process. This is where you record all of the preparation and arrangements that have been done to this point. However, you need to understand that this is only the starting line and that changes to the "Personal Long Term Care Plan" will occur along the way. For example, provisions in the care plan may change after the agreement meeting where the discussion may shed new light on the issues. Or if you are creating this plan now and may not need care for another 20 or 30 years, provisions will change as you grow older.

You also record on the "Personal Long Term Care Plan" worksheets your desires and your direction for how you want long term care services to be provided. You also indicate your preferences for living arrangements under various scenarios of long term care needs.

If you are preparing a long term care plan that may not go into effect many years from now--for example 20 or 30 years from now--you cannot be as specific in your directions as someone who is preparing a plan and receiving care currently or where the need for care is imminent. Remember to update your plan and keep it current.

This does not mean a distant future plan is any less important and that you should put off going through this exercise of planning. No one knows when the need for long term care will arise. Declaring your intentions now and sharing that with family members or other interested parties will help them immensely when they have to deal with your care in the future.

The "Personal Long Term Care Plan" worksheets beginning on page 147 are to be filled out and to remain with the book for providing a one-source reference for caregivers, care coordinators, family members and others interested in your welfare.

Organize a Care Planning and Agreement Meeting

You've done the research, gathered the documents, decided on who will be the Personal Care Coordinator and written a plan. Now it is time to present it to the family or other involved parties.

<u>This final action is the most important one.</u> If one person has been designated caregiver and wants the other persons attending the meeting to give support with respite care, transportation to doctors, etc., everyone needs to be aware of this and in total agreement to do it. All must also be willing to work with the member of the family, friend or professional who is the Personal Care Coordinator. If each attendee is given a copy of the instructions and wishes, he or she will be more understanding and supportive.

If the Personal Care Coordinator or caregiver is not a family member, it is important that the family know this and that they are willing to work with this person in support of the care.

We keep saying "IMPORTANT" as we talk about bringing the participants together. Experience has shown that even families that are close can quickly grow angry, jealous and hostile towards each other when an aging parent begins to need long term care. If a sibling moves into the parent's home, others can easily be suspicious of ulterior motives and fear to lose their inheritance. On the other hand, the child doing the entire care taking becomes bitter and feels there is no support or help from siblings.

One example of a family misunderstanding is that of a brother accusing his sister of stealing all of the money from the sale of his parent's home.

Karen, who was a single mom with two children, moved in with her parents when her father had a stroke to help her mother take care of him. Her mother was also disabled. Needing money to pay for a home care service, Karen helped her mother do a reverse mortgage on the home, which gave the needed funds. If communication had been open and Karen's brother had known the need and been involved with his parents care, he would not have reacted negatively.

Every family is different. Some families are close and some have never been compatible. Nonetheless, all family members should be invited to the agreement meeting. If you feel the communication will be strained, consider having a professional mediator present. The mediator will be able to keep things calm and running smoothly and help work out each persons concern. Make sure you get everyone's consent before bringing in a mediator.

Then--*and here is another IMPORTANT issue*--ask for each member attending to give his or her input. Allow participants to voice their concerns and give suggestions. Encourage each person to tell what he likes and dislikes about the care plan. For those who disagree, ask how they would like to see that part handled.

This does not mean you need to change your plan. The person needing the care is the ultimate decision maker. But if a small change will make everyone more supportive, it is worth it. It is very important not to dictate but to encourage attendees to communicate their concerns, their desires or their suggestions and be a part of the long term care plan.

Complete a Care Planning Agreement

GET IT IN WRITING! All good intentions seem to be forgotten with time. It may be years after this meeting before the long term care plan begins. If there are vocal commitments to help with transportation to doctors, give respite to the caregiver or other commitments, write them down on the care agreement. You can even have each person put a signature to his or her commitment if you think that is important.

This agreement form should be kept with the long term care plan in the book and a copy given to every family member. We have designed the forms to make this easy for you to do.

Here is how we suggest you conduct your meeting and get commitments on the "Care Planning Agreement" form.

The first step to holding a meeting, and perhaps the most difficult one, is to get all interested persons together in one place at one time. If it's a family gathering, perhaps a birthday, an anniversary or another special event could be used as a way to get all to meet. Or maybe even a special dinner might be an incentive.

The person conducting the meeting can be a parent or one person of a couple who are doing their planning, years before the need for care arises. A meeting on behalf of someone already receiving care or needing care in the immediate future could be conducted by that person or by a member of the family, by an adviser or a friend. The person conducting the meeting should be someone who is respected by all those attending. Preferably, this is the Care Coordinator.

The agenda could be formal or informal. If you want a formal agenda, we suggest using our care planning checklist as the agenda.

Copies of the care plan should be prepared prior to the meeting and presented to those attending. Discussion is encouraged and we recommend that the person in charge not dictate but encourage input from everyone.

After a thorough discussion of the issues and the presentation of the solutions to the problems that will be encountered, there should be a consensus of all attending to support the plan. If the plan needs to be altered to meet everyone's expectations then by all means do so if that can be done. But it is not always possible to please everyone so there must sometimes be compromise.

The end of the meeting should consist of asking everyone present to make his or her commitment to support the plan. This might just simply be moral support and agreement to abide by the provisions or it is hoped that those attending will volunteer to do something constructive. This might mean commitments to providing care, transportation, financial support, making legal arrangements or some other tangible support.

Complete the "Care Planning Agreement" form. This planning agreement is not a contract, but writing down these commitments on the agreement form is one of the most important parts of the planning process. By having a written agreement, it is more likely that those attending will fulfill their commitments.

One way to do this, that may be less offensive to some people, is to pass the agreement form around after a discussion where help is offered and ask each person to write down his or her offer of help and sign it so that the care coordinator will know whom to call later on.

If an agreement is not produced during this meeting, then an effort should be made to have additional meetings until an agreement is reached. If no agreement is eventually reached, then the plan must go forward as outlined, with the care coordinator in charge, and hopefully no major family disputes or unsolvable problems will occur.

We have provided a detachable copy of the care agreement form at the back of this book on page 159 so you can remove it to use at your meeting.

When an agreement is reached and the form filled out, be sure to transcribe the information from the detachable copy of the agreement to the permanent agreement form on page 157 in the yellow-colored section of this book. You will also want to make copies of the completed form to give to everyone who attended the meeting or who is involved in your plan.

You're finished with the formal part of the planning process. You're now ready to start implementing the care planning decisions you have made by following the agreement everyone has accepted.

PART II – LONG TERM CARE PLANNING DOCUMENTS

This section of the book contains the forms listed below. These are to be filled out in making your long term care plan. Once completed, these forms become the basis of your plan by providing those who are interested in your welfare, the information, resources and instructions necessary to carry out your wishes.

Checklist for Making a Long Term Care Plan

This is a condensed version of the information in the Part I. Use this checklist to help you understand what has to be done in preparing the "Personal Long Term Care Plan." We also provide a detachable copy of this same checklist as the very last page in this book.

___Understand there are two different care planning scenarios.
Two different categories of people need to do care planning. The first are those people who are receiving care or for whom care is imminent. The second category is those who are healthy but want to plan for care in advance in order to relieve the financial burden and stress on family or friends. Page 117

___Understand how this book becomes your care plan.
This book is designed to be a single-source reference for care provider information, for recording your personal information, for writing down the care plan and for being the repository of a written agreement. Read more on page 124.

___Fill out the "Care Planning Survey."
The survey is found in the yellow section at the back of the book, starting at page 143. Read the section about using the survey in Part I on page 125 before filling it out. The purpose of the survey is to help you determine what resources are already in place and what is missing and should be included in your plan.

___Gather information.
The survey above will help you identify resources that are necessary for a successful long term care plan. After identifying these needs you should check out the providers and advisers who can provide the necessary arrangements or services for completing the long term care plan. See page 125 for more detail.

___Choose a care coordinator.
Determining who will be a care coordinator is one of the most important parts of the plan. This person acts as a manager for arranging finances, supporting the caregivers, coordinating caregiving commitments from family or friends, paying bills, acting as a power of attorney and so on. This person is not the caregiver. See page 126 for more detail.

___Identify needed legal and end-of-life arrangements.
This action is the result of the survey and the information you gathered as a result of the survey to provide missing legal and end-of-life arrangements. You should take action to complete these missing arrangements either by having the care coordinator accomplish this or having those persons attending the agreement meeting assume some of this responsibility. You may also have to accomplish these tasks yourself. See page 128 more detail.

___Identify financial, government and provider resources.
This action is done for the same reason as the action above except arrangements are made, in this case, to identify and hopefully obtain additional financial, government and provider support for the care plan. See page 131 for more detail.

___Complete the "Personal Long Term Care Plan" worksheets.
Completing a written plan is the focus of this book. All actions up to this point have provided information and arrangements for completing the written section of the book entitled "Personal Long Term Care Plan." These 10 planning sheets are found in the yellow section of the book starting on page 147. For more information on completing this action please read page 134.

___Organize a planning and agreement meeting.
The purpose of this meeting is to explain the care plan to those persons involved with the care of a loved one. The meeting is also held to garner commitments from these people to support the care plan. See page 135 for more detail.

___Complete a care planning agreement.
A successful long term care plan will include an agreement from those people involved in the care of a loved one to provide various kinds of support. This may only include a promise to support the actions of others. Ideally, the agreement will include commitments from most persons attending the planning meeting to provide tangible support such as caregiving, transportation, financial contributions, and so on. Those people offering a commitment should sign the agreement. See page 136.

Care Planning Survey

In completing this worksheet, you will be able to spot the areas where you need to obtain more information or need to contact professional help in order to complete the long term care plan.

Your Name _____ Your Date of Birth _____

Spouse Name (if applicable) _____ Spouse DOB _____

Street Address _____

City, State, Zip _____ Phone _____

Preferences for future care providers. (In each blank, #1 to #5, #1 is highest preference.)
____ A family member will provide care, with help from other family or professionals.
____ A friend will provide care, possibly with help from professionals.
____ A home health agency or personal care agency will provide care.
____ Care will be provided by the staff of an assisted living facility.
____ Care will be provided by the staff of a nursing home.

Preferences for the future care setting in which you want your own long-term care to take place. (Put in each blank, preferences from #1 to #5, #1 being highest preference.)
____ Remain in your own home as long as possible.
____ Live with a family member or friend as long as possible.
____ Live in a retirement community or independent living complex as long as possible.
____ Live in a congregate care or assisted living facility.
____ Live in a nursing home.

Preferences for spouse's future care providers. (Put in each blank, preferences from #1 to #5, #1 being highest preference.)
____ A family member will provide care, with help from other family or professionals.
____ A friend will provide care, possibly with help from professionals.
____ A home health agency or personal care agency will provide care.
____ Care will be provided by the staff of an assisted living facility.
____ Care will be provided by the staff of a nursing home.

Preferences for the future care setting in which spouse wants long term care to take place. (Put in each blank, preferences from #1 to #5, #1 being highest preference.)
____ Remain in your own home as long as possible.
____ Live with a family member or friend as long as possible.
____ Live in a retirement community or independent living complex as long as possible.
____ Live in a congregate care or assisted living facility.
____ Live in a nursing home.

Does the care recipient have someone who can act as a Personal Care Coordinator?

Yes __ No __

(Care Planning Survey, continued)

If yes, what is the relationship of that person to you? _____

If no, have you considered the services of a Professional Care Manager? Yes__ No__

Name of Personal Care Coordinator _____
Contact info for Personal coordinator _____

In preparing to express the wishes for a personal care plan have you filled out the:
___ Instruction sheet (below) for Personal Care Coordinator (Check indicates "yes")
___ Personal and medical information recorded on instruction sheet (sheet below)

The Personal Care Coordinator will work with the current or future potential caregiver
Will the caregiver be a family member?   Yes___ No ___
Will the caregiver be a professional service provider?   Yes___ No ___
Name of caregiver_____
Address of caregiver_____
Phone number of caregiver _____

Does care recipient and/or spouse have any of the following documents?
___ Will?   For Spouse? ___   Date of last review. _____
___ Living Will? For Spouse? ___
___ A POLST form for care? Spouse? ___

Does the care recipient have any of the following documents for himself or herself?
(Check those that are applicable.)
___ General Power of Attorney
___ Springing Power of Attorney
___ Durable Power of Attorney
___ Medical Power of Attorney

Does the spouse (if it pertains) have any of the following documents for himself or
herself? (Check those that are applicable.)
___ General Power of Attorney
___ Springing Power of Attorney
___ Durable Power of Attorney
___ Medical Power of Attorney

Do anyone in the care recipient household have any of the following types of trusts?
___ Family or Living Trust   Date of last review. _____
___ Charitable Remainder Trust   Date of last review. _____
___ Generation Skipping Trust   Date of last review. _____
___ Other Trusts   Date of last review. _____

Is there a family limited partnership? Yes__ No__

Have you read in this book & understood Medicaid qualifications?   Yes ___   No ___

(Care Planning Survey, continued)

Do you need advice with strategies to lessen the financial burden of Medicaid?
Yes__ No__

Does the care recipient or family have a need requiring the advice of an elder law attorney or estate planning attorney? Yes___   No___

Does the care recipient have private insurance to pay for the cost of care?
Yes ___ No ___

Are there any other financial arrangements to pay the cost of care? Yes ___ No ___

Have you made a list of the following accounts or insurance policies for the Personal Care Coordinator?
___ Bank accounts, checking, savings, safe deposit box
___ Tax deferred savings accounts
___ Retirement funds such as pension, etc
___ Annuities and trusts
___ Life insurance policies
___ Health insurance policies
___ Long term care insurance policies
___ Medicare Insurance information
___ Other accounts for policies

_____

_____

_____

_____

Real estate assets owned by the care recipient or spouse/child living in the home
___ Personal Residence
___ 2nd Residence, cabin, rental, etc
___ Investment Property
___ Business

Do you need advice about Long Term Care Insurance? Yes___ No ___
Do you need help with Medicare Insurance, advantage plans Yes__ No__
Do you need advice from a retirement planner? Yes ___ No ___
Do you need a Senior Real Estate Specialist to consult with selling real property?
Yes ___ No ___

Are you aware of community services in your area?
___ Senior Centers
___ Senior Corps
___ Area Agencies on Aging
___ Church and community aging support groups

If the care recipient has traditional Medicare, an Advantage Plan or a prescription drug plan, do you know the benefits?
___ Inpatient Hospital
___ Nursing Home
___ Home Health Care
___ Hospice
___ Outpatient medical care
___ Drug benefits

If the care recipient is a war veteran or the surviving widow of a veteran, he or she might receive additional income to help pay for nursing home, assisted living, or home care
Do you understand the VA qualifications?   Yes ___ No ___
Do you know how to apply for benefits?   Yes ___ No ___
Do you need more information on VA benefits? Yes ___ No ___

Do you need help understanding Medicare and Medicaid Services? Yes___ No ___

Did you serve at least 90 days on active duty during a period of war, or are you the surviving spouse of such a veteran? Yes___ No ___

Review the pages in Step 1 under Community and Government Long Term Care Programs. If you still need more information or help applying for these programs we suggest you contact a professional who services that area.

Professional Long Term Care Service Providers
In Step 3 we reviewed the services of 12 professional long term care providers. You may need one or more of these services sometime during the period of care. They can save time, money, and stress in providing for long term care needs.

___ Geriatric Medical Services, Physician, Clinic, Nurses
___ Professional Care Manager
___ Professional Home Care Services
___ Home Maintenance and Chores Services
___ Home Medical Equipment and Medical Alert
___ Elder Law Advice and Estate Planning
___ Elder Mediation Services
___ Guardianship and Conservatorship
___ Financial Service Specialists
___ Senior Relocation Real Estate Specialist
___ Hospice Specialist
___ Pre-Planned Funeral Director

Personal Long Term Care Plan

Personal Information

Name_____ Date of Birth_____

Spouse's Name_____ Date of Birth_____

Marriage date_____

Copies of identification. Put certificate or ID numbers on this sheet and identify the location of the original documents

Birth Certificate_____

_____

Social Security Card_____

_____

Drivers License or ID Card_____

_____

Military ID Card_____

_____

Medical Insurance Cards_____

_____

Medicare/Medicaid Cards_____

_____

Drug Prescription Cards_____

_____

Marriage License/Certificate_____

_____

(Personal Long Term Care Plan, continued)

Medicare/Medicaid Information

Name of Advisor/Caseworker_____

Phone Number of Advisor/Caseworker_____

Address of office_____

Location of Copies of Medicaid Forms/Applications_____

_____

List and location of other important personal documents

_____

_____

_____

_____

_____

_____

_____

_____

_____

_____

_____

_____

_____

_____

_____

_____

_____

_____

_____

_____

_____

(Personal Long Term Care Plan, continued)

Care Instructions

Name of Care Coordinator_____

Address_____

Phone number(s)_____

Name of Caregiver_____

Address_____

Phone number (s)_____

Name and phone number of State Aging Services_____

_____

_____

Name and phone number of Local Aging Services_____

_____

_____

Name, address and phone number(s) of Medical Doctor(s)_____

_____

_____

_____

_____

_____

_____

Name and phone number of emergency aid_____

_____

Name and phone numbers of Home Health Agencies, Nursing Homes and other
services_____

_____

_____

_____

_____

(Personal Long Term Care Plan, continued)

Personal Information:

Health problems _____

_____

_____

_____

_____

_____

_____

_____

_____

_____

_____

_____

_____

Medications_____

_____

_____

_____

_____

_____

_____

Funeral arrangements or requests_____

_____

_____

_____

_____

_____

_____

_____

_____

_____

(Personal Long Term Care Plan, continued)

Care Instructions_____

_____

_____

_____

_____

_____

_____

_____

_____

_____

_____

_____

_____

_____

_____

_____

_____

_____

_____

_____

_____

_____

_____

_____

_____

_____

_____

_____

(Personal Long Term Care Plan, continued)

Financial Information

Record account numbers, policy numbers, and location.

Bank name and address _____

_____

_____

Checking account numbers _____

_____

_____

Savings account numbers _____

_____

_____

IRA's, Annuities, CD's _____

_____

_____

_____

_____

Security deposit box _____

_____

Income – where from and amounts _____

_____

_____

_____

_____

Other Assets _____

_____

_____

_____

_____

Insurance--List companies, policy numbers, who is insured, beneficiaries, location of documents, and when the coverage renews, if applicable.

Health Insurance Policies_____

_____

_____

_____

_____

_____

Long Term Care Insurance Policies_____

_____

_____

_____

_____

_____

Life Insurance Policies_____

_____

_____

_____

_____

_____

_____

_____

Annuities_____

_____

_____

_____

_____

_____

_____

Estate Planning Documents--Record name, date of documents and location of documents.

Copy of Will and/or Trusts_____

_____

_____

_____

General or Durable Powers of Attorney (include medical powers of attorney)

_____

_____

_____

_____

_____

Living Will_____

_____

_____

_____

Medical Treatment Plan - POLST_____

_____

_____

_____

Other Special Trusts _____

_____

_____

_____

_____

_____

(Personal Long Term Care Plan, continued)

Other Documents--Record dates, names and location of documents.

Deeds and Titles_____

_____

_____

_____

Contracts_____

_____

_____

_____

Insurance Declarations_____

_____

_____

_____

Certificates/Bonds_____

_____

_____

_____

Other Important Documents_____

_____

_____

_____

_____

_____

Who-Gets-What-List

This list is intended as an addendum to the will. We recommend putting the list here instead of putting it with the will. It should also go here if there is no will. The list belongs here because long term care is often the final event of a person's life and often robs that person of the ability to make decisions about what family members should get. In addition, the type of planning that goes into preparing for long term care would naturally include provisions for dividing up personal possessions even before death occurs. This makes inclusion here the most logical place.

This list should include those personal items of little intrinsic value, but of great sentimental value to members of the family. This would be things such as needlework, knitting projects, crochet projects, special China settings, memorabilia, journals, personal artwork, handicrafts and much more. The list should name the item and then name the person who will get it.

_____
_____
_____
_____
_____
_____
_____
_____
_____
_____
_____
_____
_____
_____
_____
_____
_____
_____
_____
_____
_____

Care Planning Agreement

Date and place of this agreement _____

List below the names of all those persons attending. If any of these persons is not a family member or friend, indicate the reason for this person attending.

_____
_____
_____
_____
_____
_____
_____
_____
_____
_____
_____
_____
_____
_____

Write in the space below and in the space on the next page, the commitments made by those attending this meeting, who have agreed to help with the long term care plan. Do this by writing the person's name followed by a description of the commitment that person has made. Be specific and provide details to include the amount of commitment, how often, when, where and so on. Or another way to do this is to have the person making a commitment personally write his or her promise on this form and possibly include his or her signature.

_____
_____
_____
_____
_____
_____
_____
_____

After this agreement is completed, make copies of both sides and send these copies to the people who attended the meeting. We have provided a duplicate copy of this form on page 159 that is perforated and can be torn out of the blook. You can transcribe the information on this form to that form to make it easier to copy or you can do the reverse--use the detachable copy for the original agreement and transcribe that information to this copy that must remain in the book. It is very important to keep a copy of the completed agreement in this book.

Care Planning Agreement (duplicate tear-out copy)
(This is a duplicate, perforated copy to be torn out of this book.)

Date and place of this agreement _____

List below the names of all those persons attending. If any of these persons is not a family member or friend, indicate the reason for this person attending.

_____

_____

_____

_____

_____

_____

_____

_____

_____

_____

_____

_____

_____

_____

Write in the space below and in the space on the next page, the commitments made by those attending this meeting, who have agreed to help with the long term care plan. Do this by writing the person's name followed by a description of the commitment that person has made. Be specific and provide details to include the amount of commitment, how often, when, where and so on. Or another way to do this is to have the person making a commitment personally write his or her promise on this form and possibly include his or her signature.

_____

_____

_____

_____

_____

_____

_____

_____

_____

_____

_____

_____

_____

_____

_____

_____

_____

_____

_____

_____

_____

_____

_____

_____

_____

_____

_____

_____

_____

_____

_____

_____

After this agreement is completed, make copies of both sides and send these copies to those people who attended the meeting. We have provided a permanent copy of this form on page 157 that is intended to remain in the book and to contain all of the information in the agreement. Make sure to transcribe all of the agreement to page 157. <u>It is very important to keep a copy of the completed agreement in this book.</u>

Checklist for Making a Long Term Care Plan (tear-out copy)
(This is a duplicate, perforated copy to be torn out of this book.)

This is a condensed version of the information in the Part I. Use this checklist to help you understand what has to be done in preparing the Personal Long Term Care Plan. We also provide a permanent copy of this same checklist on page 141.

____**Understand there are two different care planning scenarios.**
Two different categories of people need to do care planning. The first are those people who are receiving care or for whom care is imminent. The second category is those who are healthy but want to plan for care in advance in order to relieve the financial burden and stress on family or friends. See page 117 for more detail.

____**Understand how this book becomes your care plan.**
This book is designed to be a single-source reference for care provider information, for recording your personal information, for writing down the care plan and for being the repository of a written agreement. Read more on page 124.

____**Fill out the "Care Planning Survey."**
The survey is found in the yellow section at the back of the book, starting at page 143. Read the section about using the survey in Part I on page 125 before filling it out. The purpose of the survey is to help you determine what resources are already in place and what is missing and should be included in your plan.

____**Gather information.**
The survey above will help you identify resources that are necessary for a successful long term care plan. After identifying these needs you should check out the providers and advisers who can provide the necessary arrangements or services for completing the long term care plan. See page 125 for more detail.

____**Choose a care coordinator.**
Determining who will be a care coordinator is one of the most important parts of the plan. This person acts as a manager for arranging finances, supporting the caregivers, coordinating caregiving commitments from family or friends, paying bills, acting as a power of attorney and so on. This person is not the caregiver. See page 126 for more detail.

___**Identify needed legal and end-of-life arrangements**.

This action is the result of the survey and the information you gathered as a result of the survey to provide missing legal and end-of-life arrangements. You should take action to complete these missing arrangements either by having the care coordinator accomplish this or having those persons attending the agreement meeting assume some of this responsibility. You may also have to accomplish these tasks yourself. See page 128 more detail.

___**Identify financial, government and provider resources.**

This action is done for the same reason as the action above except arrangements are made, in this case, to identify and hopefully obtain additional financial, government and provider support for the care plan. See page 131 for more detail.

___**Complete the "Personal Long Term Care Plan" worksheets.**

Completing a written plan is the focus of this book. All actions up to this point have provided information and arrangements for completing the written section of the book entitled "Personal Long Term Care Plan." These 10 planning sheets are found in the yellow section of the book starting on page 147. For more information on completing this action please read page 134.

___**Organize a planning and agreement meeting.**

The purpose of this meeting is to explain the care plan to those persons involved with the care of a loved one. The meeting is also held to garner commitments from these people to support the care plan. See page 135 for more detail.

___**Complete a care planning agreement.**

A successful long term care plan will include an agreement from those people involved in the care of a loved one to provide various kinds of support. This may only include a promise to support the actions of others. Ideally, the agreement will include commitments from most persons attending the planning meeting to provide tangible support such as caregiving, transportation, financial contributions, and so on. Those people offering a commitment should sign the agreement. See page 136.